LPN

PEARLS OF WISDOM

Sheryl L. Gossman
William G. Gossman
Dorothy Thompson

NOTE

The intent of *LPN Pearls of Wisdom* is to serve as a study aid to improve performance on a standardized exam. It is not intended to be a source text of the knowledge base of the nursing field, or to serve as a reference in any way for the practice of clinical nursing. Neither Boston Medical Publishing Corporation, nor the editors warrant that the information in this text is complete or accurate. The reader is encouraged to verify each answer in several references. All drug use indications and dosages must be verified by the reader before administration of any compound.

Printed by Mount Auburn Press/IKON Office Solutions, Watertown, MA.

Art Director: Maryse Charette

This book was produced using Times and Symbols fonts and computer based graphics with Macintosh® computers.

ISBN: 1-58409-002-2

DEDICATION

To our daughters Casey and Taylor.

Sheryl L. Gossman

William G. Gossman

To my grandmother, Pearl, for without her, there would be no me.

Dorothy Thompson

AUTHORS AND EDITORS

Sheryl L. Gossman, RN, BSN
Naperville, IL

William G. Gossman, M.D., FAAEM
Project Medical Director
Mount Sinai Medical Center
Chicago, IL

Dorothy Thomspon, LPN
St. Anthony's Hospital
St. Petersburg, FL

ASSOCIATE EDITORS

Brent Grady, RN, CCRN, CEN
Assistant Nurse Manager
Department of Emergency Medicine
Mount Sinai Medical Center
Chicago, IL

Kwesi Hankins, RN
Department of Emergency Medicine
Illinois Masonic Medical Center
Chicago, IL

Kathryn McGinnis, RN, BSN
Department of Emergency Medicine
Illinois Masonic Medical Center
Chicago, IL

Brian Murphy, RN
Critical Care Department
Little Company of Mary Hospital
Evergreen Park, IL

Anna Maria Pena, MS, RN/CS, FNP
Sinai Family Medicine
Miles Square Health Center
Chicago, IL

Kristine Wengel, RN, BSN, CCRN
Surgical Intensive Care Unit
Rush-Presbyterian-St. Luke's Medical Center
Chicago, IL

Marilyn L. Yucaitis, RNBA, CEN, TNCCP, ENPC
Department of Emergency Medicine
Mount Sinai Medical Center
Chicago, IL

CONTRIBUTING AUTHORS

Bobby Abrams, M.D.
Attending Physician
Macomb Hospital

Jonathan Adler, M.D.
Instructor of Medicine
Harvard Medical School
Boston, MA

David F.M. Brown, M.D.
Instructor in Medicine
Harvard Medical School
Massachusetts General Hospital
Boston, MA

Eduardo Castro, M.D.
Instructor in Medicine
Harvard Medical School
Massachusetts General Hospital
Boston, MA

C. James Corrall, M.D., M.P.H.
Clinical Associate Professor of Pediatrics
Clinical Associate Professor of Emergency Medicine
Indiana University School of Medicine
Indianapolis, MA

Peter Emblad, M.D.
Boston City Hospital
Boston, MS

Craig Feied, M.D.
Clinical Associate Professor
George Washington University
Washington Hospital Center

James F. Holmes, M.D.
University of California, Davis
School of Medicine
Sacramento, California

Eddie Hooker, M.D.
Assistant Professor
University of Louisville
Louisville, KY

John A. Jarboe, RN
Saint-Anthony's Hospital
Saint-Petersburg, FL

Lance W. Kreplick, M.D.
Assistant Professor
University of Illinois
EHS Christ Hospital
Oak Lawn, IL

Bernard Lopez, M.D.
Assistant Professor
Thomas Jefferson Medical College
Thomas Jefferson University Hospital
Philadelphia, PA

Gillian Lewke, P.A., C.M.A.
Physician Assistant
Westlake Hospital
Melrose Park, IL

Mary Nan S. Mallory, M.D.
Clinical Instructor
University of Louisville
Louisville, KY

David Morgan, M.D.
University of Texas
Southwestern Medical Center
Parkland Memorial Hospital
Dallas, TX

Edward A. Panacek, M.D.
Associate Professor
University of California, Davis
School of Medicine
Sacramento, CA

Scott H. Plantz, M.D.
Assistant Professor
Chicago Medical School
Mt. Sinai Medical Center
Chicago, IL

Carlo Rosen, M.D.
Instructor in Medicine
Harvard Medical School
Massachusetts General Hospital
Boston, MA

William A. Schwer, M.D.
Professor and Chairman
Rush-Presbyterian-St. Luke's Medical Center
Chicago, IL

Dana Stearns, M.D.
Instructor in Medicine
Harvard Medical School
Massachusetts General Hospital
Boston, MA

Jack Stump, M.D.
Attending Physician
Rogue Valley Medical Center
Medford, OR

Joan Surdukowski, M.D.
Assistant Professor
Chicago Medical School
Mt. Sinai Medical Center
Chicago, IL

Loire Swischer, M.D.
Assistant Professor
Allegheny University of the Health Sciences
Philadelphia, PA

WE APPRECIATE YOUR COMMENTS!

We appreciate your opinion and encourage you to send us any suggestions or recommendations. Please let us know if you discover any errors, or if there is any way we can make our LPN PEARLS OF WISDOM Text more helpful to you. We are also interested in recruiting new authors and editors. Please call, write, fax, or e-mail. We look forward to hearing from you.

S.L.G. , W.G.G., & D.T.

Return to:

Boston Medical Publishing Corporation
237 S. 70th Street, Suite 206, Lincoln, NE

1-888-MBOARDS (626-2737)
TEL.: 402-484-6118
FAX: 402-484-6552
E-mail: bmp@emedicine.com

INTRODUCTION

Congratulations! You are now entering the final phase of your nursing education - preparing to take the LPN licensure examination. Most nursing students look upon this exam with extreme anxiety and frustration. How can one possibly learn all that is necessary to pass this exam? This book is a good step towards that process. *LPN Pearls of Wisdom* has been designed to help you improve your performance on the exam as well as help you identify some weak areas in your nursing knowledge. The format of this book is different than most of the common preparation review books in that you are not asked to select the best answer. Instead the answer is provided for you. We have found that this method of board exam review will give you the basic concepts necessary for passing the exam.

How can this book help you prepare for this exam? *Pearls* is intended to serve as a study aid to improve performance on the LPN exam. To achieve this goal, the text is divided into the 4 major areas of nursing study: Medical Surgical, Maternal-Infant, Pediatrics, and Mental Heath. Incorporated into these areas are the aspects that are covered on theLPN exam. The questions are written in a straight forward question/answer format and no intention has been made to mislead or "trick" the student. The answer provided will be the best possible answer for that question.

Unlike the LPN exam, in which the answers given to a question may describe 4 different situations and you are to pick the <u>best</u>, this book looks at the underlying theory or idea behind the answer. For example, if a question is asked to determine the student's knowledge of the ABC's of resuscitation, the LPN exam will list 4 actions that could be undertaken, all of which would be appropriate within the care of an unconscious patient. However, in determining which action should be taken first, the student should understand the principles of the ABC's of resuscitation and choose an answer related to determining and maintaining the airway. It is our intent that if the student understands the premise behind the answer, any list of situations can be asked, but the student will understand which situation is in line with the correct nursing theory. Therefore, this book should be an invaluable aid in determining your basic knowledge of nursing theories and medical facts.

In order to use this book to the fullest potential, the student should go through each question using a 3x5 card to cover the answer first in order to test his/her own knowledge. If upon reading the answer you do not understand the premise behind the answer - LOOK IT UP! Information that you will learn in response to seeking the answer will be more effectively retained than merely memorizing the correct answer without understanding the rationale behind it. Check boxes have been provided for your convenience to check-off previously missed or answered questions, whichever is your preference.

Pearls is an interactive book designed to be used many times over. Test your knowledge by going through the book more that once and learn from your mistakes. Using this book in a group setting may also be helpful. Each individual in the group could determine their answer and then as a group compare. If there are discrepancies, look up the answer and determine why the answer is correct or incorrect.

Great care has been to taken to determine the best possible questions and answers needed to pass the LPN exam. Some questions and answers may seem outdated, however we have attempted to form the questions so they are an accurate representation of those found on the exam. As always, we welcome your comments regarding questions, content, and any improvements or suggestions.

Study hard and good luck!

S.L.G., W.G.G., & D.T.

TABLE OF CONTENTS

MEDICAL-SURGICAL PEARLS 9

MATERNAL-INFANT PEARLS 149

PEDIATRIC PEARLS 206

MENTAL HEALTH PEARLS 274

BIBLIOGRAPHY 309

MEDICAL - SURGICAL PEARLS

"Extreme remedies are very appropriate for severe diseases."
Hippocrates

❐❐ **How should the hair surrounding a wound be removed prior to wound repair?**

By clipping, as razor removal will increase the infection rate.

❐❐ **When should a nasal gastric tube be pulled?**

When ordered by the physician.

❐❐ **What technique should be used to insert a Foley catheter?**

Sterile.

❐❐ **How can you confirm placement of a Foley catheter?**

When you see urine return in the tube.

❐❐ **T/F: 30 ez. equal 1 cc.**

False. 30 cc equal 1 oz.

❐❐ **A condition in which the blood vessels lose their elasticity known as "hardening of the arteries," is also known as what?**

Arteriosclerosis.

❐❐ **How long can wound care be delayed before proliferation of bacteria (which may result in infection) occurs?**

3 hours.

❐❐ **Which factors increase the likelihood of wound infection?**

Infection rate is increased if the wound is dirty or contaminated, stellate or crushing, longer than 5 cm, older than 6 hours, and/or if the wound's location is an infection prone anatomic site.

❐❐ **What types of wounds result in the majority of tetanus cases?**

Lacerations, punctures, and crush injuries.

❐❐ **What is the most likely cause of fever in a patient who has had surgery within the past 48 hours?**

Atelectasis.

❑❑ T/F: In general, women live longer than men do.

True.

❑❑ What is the most likely cause of fever in a patient who is 5-7 days postoperative?

Wound infection.

❑❑ Which common electrolyte disturbances occur in patients who have acute pancreatitis?

Hypocalcemia and hypomagnesemia.

❑❑ Define autonomy.

Self governance or not being controlled by outside forces or individuals.

❑❑ Match the following transplant types with their definitions.

Autograft	a. Donor and recipient are genetically the same.
Heterotrophic	b. Donor and recipient are the same person.
Isograft	c. Donor and recipient are of the same species.
Orthotopic	d. Donor and recipient belong to different species.
Allograft	e. Transplantation to a normal anatomical position.
Xenograft	f. Transplantation to a different anatomical position.

Answers: 1: b, 2: f, 3: a, 4: e, 5: c, 6: d.

❑❑ If a patient has been burned over his entire back, both legs, and right arm, what percentage of his body is considered to be burned?

63%. Burn percentages are calculated through the rule of 9's:
Face : 9%
Arms : 9% each
Front : 18%
Back : 18%
Legs : 18% each

❑❑ Which type of hemorrhoids are most painful, internal or external?

External. Internal hemorrhoids have a nerve supply from the autonomic nervous system, which has no sensory fibers. The nerve supply for external hemorrhoids is supplied by the inferior rectal nerve and does have sensory fibers, thereby increasing the pain.

❑❑ What preventative measures would you suggest for the treatment of hemorrhoids?

A high fiber diet, sitz baths, and good hygiene.

❑❑ Torsion of the testicles is most common in which age group?

Adolescents.

❒❒ **What is the maximal amount of time that a testes can remain torsed without irreversible damage being done?**

4–6 hours.

❒❒ **Where in the brain is the respiratory control center?**

Medulla oblongata.

❒❒ **Which drug reverses heparin after open heart surgery?**

Protamine.

❒❒ **If oxygen is withheld or cut off, death will occur in how long?**

4-6 minutes.

❒❒ **How long can the brain survive without oxygen?**

3 minutes.

❒❒ **External respiration is known by what other name?**

Ventilation.

❒❒ **What are some possible causes of distended neck veins in a trauma patient?**

Tension pneumothorax, pericardial tamponade, air embolism, and cardiac failure. Neck vein distention may not be present until hypovolemia has been treated.

❒❒ **What life threatening injury is associated with pelvic fractures?**

Severe hemorrhage, usually retroperitoneal. Up to 6 liters of blood can be accommodated in this space.

❒❒ **What is a stress fracture?**

A stress or "fatigue" fracture is caused by small, repetitive forces, usually involving the metatarsal shafts, the distal tibia, or the femoral neck. These fractures may not be seen on initial radiographs.

❒❒ **What is nursemaid's elbow?**

Subluxation of the radial head. During forceful retraction, some fibers of the annular ligament, which encircles the radial neck, become trapped between the radial head and the capitellum. The arm is usually in slight flexion and pronation.

❒❒ **What is compartment syndrome?**

Increased pressure within closed tissue spaces, which compromises blood flow to muscle and nerve tissue. Contributing causes include external compression (by burn eschar, circumferential casts, dressings, or pneumatic pressure garments), and volume increase within the compartment (due to hemorrhage into the compartment, IV infiltration, or edema with post-ischemic swelling that is secondary to injury).

❒❒ What are the early signs and symptoms of compartment syndrome?

Tenderness and pain out of proportion to the injury, pain that accompanies active and passive motion, and hypesthesia (paresthesia) with an abnormal, 2-point discrimination.

❒❒ Name the late signs and symptoms of compartment syndrome.

Compartment is tense, indurated, and erythematous, there is pallor and pulselessness, and capillary refill is slow.

❒❒ Acute tinnitus is associated with toxicity of which medication?

Salicylates. Other causes of tinnitus include vascular abnormalities, mechanical abnormalities, and damaged cochlear hair cells. Unilateral tinnitus is associated with trauma, chronic suppurative otitis, and Meniere's disease.

❒❒ In giving intravenous fluids, you are responsible for ensuring that your patient gets the right amount, correct rate, and proper solution. Before giving any medication or solution, you should check for what?

Correct patient, amount, dosage, route, and time.

❒❒ What methods can be used for the emergency storage of an avulsed tooth?

The tooth can be placed in a small container of milk, or the patient may place the tooth underneath his/her tongue.

❒❒ A 47- year-old female complains of an excruciating waxing and waning "electric shock type" pain in her right cheek. What syndrome is commonly associated with this type of pain?

Tic douloureux. The most significant finding is that the pain follows the distribution of the trigeminal nerve. Minor trigger zone stimulation can consistently reproduce the pain.

❒❒ Where would rods and cones be found?

Mainly around the periphery of the retina.

❒❒ When should a patient's eye not be dilated?

When the patient has narrow angle glaucoma or an iris-supported intraocular lens.

❒❒ Why shouldn't a patient use topical ophthalmologic anesthetics on a regular basis?

These anesthetics inhibit healing and eliminate sensation, thereby decreasing the eye's natural ability to protect itself.

❒❒ What physical findings suggest an acute aortic dissection?

BP differences between arms and/or legs, cardiac tamponade, and aortic insufficiency murmur.

❑❑ **Name some common Valsalva maneuvers.**

Holding the breath, stimulation of the gag reflex, squatting, pressure on the eyeball, or immersing the face in ice.

❑❑ **What are some of the adverse effects of lidocaine?**

Drowsiness, nausea, vertigo, confusion, ataxia, tinnitus, muscle twitching, respiratory depression, and psychosis.

❑❑ **Before you administer any pain medication, for what should you check?**

When any previous pain medication was given and recent vital signs.

❑❑ **When administering CPR, what is the ventilation to compression ratio for one rescuer?**

2 breaths to 15 compressions.

❑❑ **What is the ventilation to compression ratio for 2 rescuers?**

1 breath to 5 compressions.

❑❑ **The CDC defines how many categories of specific isolation?**

There are 7 categories:
- Respiratory isolation.
- Drainage/secretion precaution.
- Blood/body fluid precaution.
- Strict isolation.
- Contact isolation.
- AFB (TB) isolation.
- Enteric precaution

❑❑ **What is the difference between isolation and precaution?**

Isolation requires a private room. Precaution does not.

❑❑ **Which hypertensive medications should not be administered to diabetics?**

Diuretics and b-blockers. These drugs increase insulin resistance. ACE inhibitors are the drugs of choice for these patients.

❑❑ **What is the most common side effect of b-blockers?**

Fatigue, which occurs early in treatment; and depression, which occurs later.

❑❑ **You are at a restaurant, and a woman at the next table next begins to cough loudly. She stands up and begins wheezing between coughs, but is still able to speak. How should you help her?**

Encourage her to cough deeper. Do not interrupt her own spontaneous attempts at expulsion if she still has good air exchange. However, should she begin to display severe respiratory difficulty with a weakening cough and the inability to talk, the Heimlich maneuver should be initiated.

❑❑ One of your patients is diagnosed as obese. What is the definition of obesity?

An excess of body fat, generally 20% above the ideal body weight.

❑❑ The normal Heimlich maneuver is not very effective on people who are pregnant or markedly obese. What should be done for these individuals when they are in severe respiratory distress?

Position your fists above the person's navel, place your cupped fist on the chest, and deliver swift thrusts.

❑❑ T/F: Most falls occur in the home.

True.

❑❑ Asbestosis is associated with an increased risk of what 2 diseases?

Lung cancer and malignant mesothelioma.

❑❑ What procedures should be performed to confine aspiration in a patient who is continuously vomiting and at risk for aspiration pneumonia?

Lie the patient on his right side in the Trendelenburg position. This will help confine the aspiration to the right upper lobe.

❑❑ What conditions will most likely be found in the family history of asthmatic patients?

Asthma, allergies, and/or atopic dermatitis.

❑❑ What is the most common postoperative respiratory complication?

Atelectasis. Respiratory failure and aspiration pneumonia are other postoperative complications.

❑❑ What are the 5 risk factors of cancer?

Cigarette smoking.
High fat diet.
Salt cured, smoked, nitrite-cured foods.
Excessive alcohol intake.
Excessive exposure to the sun.

❑❑ Other than smoking, name some risk factors for COPD.

Environmental pollutants, recurrent upper respiratory infections (especially in infancy), eosinophilia or increased serum IgE, bronchial hyper-responsiveness, a family history of COPD, and protease deficiencies.

❑❑ Is there any hope for patients with COPD, if they quit smoking?

Yes. Symptomatically speaking, coughing stops in up to 80% of these patients. 54% of COPD patients find relief within one month after quitting.

❒❒ **Your vitamin-crazed father insists that his daily dose of vitamin C has helped him avoid colds for the past 53 years. Is there any validity to his statement?**

No. Studies have failed to show that vitamin C has any prophylactic effects. However, studies suggested that consuming 1 g of vitamin C a day can decreases the severity and duration of the symptoms associated with the common cold.

❒❒ **T/F: Vitamin D deficiency results in normal bone formation in infants.**

False.

❒❒ **Define range of motion.**

Methods of exercising the joints to prevent contractions and to stimulate circulation.

❒❒ **T/F: In a 4-point gait the patient bears weight on one leg.**

False.

❒❒ **Name the most common types of gait.**

Four-point, 2-point, swing through, and swing to gait.

❒❒ **T/F: Vitamin E deficiency usually does not manifest as hemolytic anemia in low-birth-weight or premature infants.**

False.

❒❒ **Infants born to iodine-deficient mothers may be born with what disease?**

Cretinism.

❒❒ **T/F: During the period of rapid growth, children are susceptible to the deficiency of zinc.**

True.

❒❒ **T/F: Staphylococcus aureus is the most common isolated orgasm found in infected surgical wounds.**

True.

❒❒ **Define a compromised host.**

A person with a deficient defense mechanism.

❒❒ **What age group is afflicted with the most colds per year?**

Kindergartners, who have an average of 12 colds per year. Second place goes to preschoolers, who average 6 -10 per year. School children catch an average of 7 per year, and adolescents and adults average only 2-4 per year.

❒❒ **How long, on average, does the common cold last?**

3-10 days.

❒❒ **What is the most common presentation of cystic fibrosis in newborns?**

GI obstruction, which is due to meconium ileus.

❒❒ **Are aspirated foreign bodies more likely to be found in the right or left bronchus?**

The right. This is because the right bronchus is straighter, and foreign objects are more likely to follow this path.

❒❒ **A patient complaining of chronic hoarseness is scheduled for a laryngoscopy. What disease is the M.D. looking to rule out?**

If hoarseness lasts for more than 4–6 weeks, this examination should be performed to eliminate the possibility of laryngeal carcinoma.

❒❒ **What is the most common type of cancer in the U.S.?**

Lung cancer, which is also the leading cause of death.

❒❒ **Define metastasis.**

Malignant cells break away from the original sites and are transported by the lymph or blood to a new site.

❒❒ **Sarcoma arise from what type of tissue?**

Connective tissue.

❒❒ **Sarcoma and carcinoma are referred to as what type of tumors?**

Solid tumors.

❒❒ **What disease is associated with infections such as PCP, TB, histoplasmosis, cryptococcus and CMV?**

HIV.

❒❒ **What percentage of PE's are caused by DVT's?**

95%.

❒❒ **After the fracture of a long or pelvic bone, you should assess for what type of embolism?**

Fat.

❑❑ **What are some of the signs and symptoms of a fat embolism?**

Dyspnea, copious production of thick white sputum, tachycardia, and wheezing.

❑❑ **What are the classic signs and symptoms of TB?**

Night sweats, fever, weight loss, malaise, cough, and a greenish-yellow sputum most commonly seen in the mornings.

❑❑ **Where are some common extrapulmonary TB sites?**

The lymph node, bone, GI tract, GU tract, meninges, liver, and the pericardium.

❑❑ **Lymph node function is related to what system?**

Immune system.

❑❑ **Which electrolyte imbalances might be present in a cirrhotic patient who presents with weakness and edema?**

Hyponatremia (dilutional or diuretic-induced), hypokalemia (from GI losses, secondary hyperaldosteronism, or diuretics), and hypomagnesemia.

❑❑ **What are the current recommendations from the American Cancer Society for screening colon cancer?**

An annual digital exam for patients over 40 and an annual testing for occult blood in patients over 50. A flexible sigmoidoscopy should be performed every 3-5 years on individuals older than 50 years. Earlier screening is required in patients with familial polyposis.

❑❑ **What is the most common cause of cellulitis?**

An infection with Streptococcus pyogenes or Staphylococcus aureus without a break in the skin.

❑❑ **What are the major signs and symptoms of cellulitis?**

Local redness, swelling, and tenderness at the site.

❑❑ **What is the most common cause of bacterial diarrhea?**

E. coli (enteroinvasive, enteropathogenic, enterotoxigenic).

❑❑ **Which is the most common form of acute diarrhea?**

Viral diarrhea. It is generally self-limited, lasting only 1-3 days.

❑❑ **What is the most probable cause of diarrhea that develops within 12 hours of a meal?**

An ingested pre-formed toxin.

❑❑ **When does traveler's diarrhea typically occur?**

3-7 days after arrival in a foreign land.

❑❑ **What is the definition of chronic diarrhea?**

The passage of greater than 200 g of loose stool per day for over 3 weeks.

❑❑ **What physical findings would make you suspect that a child has swallowed a foreign body?**

Besides the child's distress, dysphagia, a high fever, peritoneal signs, and a red or scratched oropharynx may be evident. In addition, subcutaneous air suggests perforation.

❑❑ **You stick yourself with a needle from a chronic hepatitis B carrier. You've been vaccinated, but have never had your antibody status checked. What is the appropriate post exposure prophylaxis?**

Measure your anti-HB's titer. If it is adequate (> 10 mIU), treatment is not required. If it is inadequate, you'll need a vaccine booster and a single dose of HBIG as soon as possible.

❑❑ **What syndrome is indicated by crampy abdominal pain and mucus-filled stool?**

Irritable bowel syndrome. Patients are afebrile and often improve after passing flatus.

❑❑ **Hayfever is an example of what?**

Autoimmune sensitivity.

❑❑ **List 4 contraindications to the introduction of a nasogastric tube.**

Suspected esophageal laceration or perforation, near obstruction due to stricture, esophageal foreign body, and severe head trauma with rhinorrhea.

❑❑ **When is a person considered obese?**

An individual with an average weight 20% above the weight recommended for their height is considered obese.

❑❑ **What are the major causes of acute pancreatitis?**

Alcohol and biliary stone disease.

❑❑ **Epigastric pain that radiates to the back and is relieved, to some extent, by sitting up is indicative of what disease?**

Pancreatitis.

❑❑ **T/F: Movement of water through the capillary wall is unrestricted.**

True.

❑❑ **How does hyperglycemia lead to hyponatremia?**

Because glucose stays in the extracellular fluid, hyperglycemia draws water out of the cell into the extracellular fluid. Each 100 mg/dL increase in plasma glucose decreases the serum sodium by 1.6 to 1.8 mEq/L.

❑❑ **What are the signs and symptoms of hyponatremia?**

Weakness, nausea, anorexia, vomiting, confusion, lethargy, seizures, and coma.

❑❑ **What are the most common causes of the hypotonic fluid loss which leads to hypernatremia?**

Diarrhea, vomiting, hyperpyrexia, and excessive sweating.

❑❑ **What are the signs and symptoms of hypernatremia?**

Confusion, muscle irritability, seizures, respiratory paralysis, and coma.

❑❑ **What are the monitor findings on a patient with hypokalemia?**

Flattened T-waves, depressed ST segments, prominent P-waves, prominent U-waves, and prolonged QT and PR intervals.

❑❑ **What are the monitor findings on a patient with hyperkalemia?**

Peaked T-waves, prolonged QT and PR intervals, diminished P-waves, depressed T-waves, QRS widening, levels exceeding 10 mEq/L, and a classic sine wave.

❑❑ **What is the first monitor finding for a patient with hyperkalemia?**

The development of tall-peaked T-waves at levels of 5.6–6.0 mEq/L, which are best seen in the precordial leads.

❑❑ **What are the causes of hyperkalemia?**

Acidosis, tissue necrosis, hemolysis, blood transfusions, GI bleed, renal failure, Addison's disease, primary hypoaldosteronism, excess po K+ intake, RTA IV, and medications such as succinylcholine, b-blockers, captopril (Capoten), spironolactone, triamterene, amiloride, and high dose penicillin.

❑❑ **What are the causes of hypocalcemia?**

Shock, sepsis, multiple blood transfusions, hypoparathyroidism, vitamin D deficiency, pancreatitis, hypomagnesemia, alkalosis, fat embolism syndrome, phosphate overload, chronic renal failure, loop diuretics, hypoalbuminemia, tumor lysis syndrome, and medication, such as Dilantin, phenobarbital, heparin, theophylline, cimetidine, and gentamicin.

❑❑ **What is the most common cause of hyperkalemia?**

Chronic renal failure is the most common cause of "true hyperkalemia."

❑❑ **What are the most common causes of hypercalcemia?**

In descending order: malignancy, primary hyperparathyroidism, and thiazide diuretics.

❑❑ What are the signs and symptoms of hypercalcemia?

The most common gastrointestinal symptoms are anorexia and constipation. A classic mnemonic can be used to remember them:

- Stones: renal calculi.
- Bones: osteolysis.
- Abdominal groans: peptic ulcer disease and pancreatitis.
- Psychic overtones: psychiatric disorders.

❑❑ T/F: Most causes of acute cholecystitis are caused by gallstones lodged in the cystic duct.

True.

❑❑ What would be one of the diagnostic tests ordered for your patient suspected to have cholecyslitis?

Sonography to visualize stones.

❑❑ What is the initial treatment for hypercalcemia?

Patients with hypercalcemia are dehydrated because high calcium levels interfere with ADH and the ability of the kidney to concentrate urine. Therefore, the initial treatment is restoration of the extracellular fluid with 5-10 L of normal saline within 24 hours. After the patient is rehydrated, administer Furosemide in doses of 1-3 mg/kg.

❑❑ What is the most common cause of hyperphosphatemia?

Acute and chronic renal failure.

❑❑ What are the signs and symptoms of primary adrenal insufficiency?

Fatigue, weakness, weight loss, anorexia, hyperpigmentation, nausea, vomiting, abdominal pain, diarrhea, and orthostatic hypotension.

❑❑ What lab findings are associated with primary adrenal insufficiency?

Hyperkalemia, hyponatremia, hypoglycemia, azotemia (if volume depletion is present), and a mild metabolic acidosis.

❑❑ What causes acute adrenal crisis?

It occurs secondary to a major stress, such as surgery, severe injury, myocardial infarction, or any other illness in a patient with primary or secondary adrenal insufficiency.

❑❑ T/F: The chemical name for aspirin is acetylsalicylic acid.

True.

❑❑ What are some of the signs and symptoms of aspirin toxicity?

Rapid breathing, vomiting, headache, irritability, and hypoglycemia.

❑❑ Your patient has a diagnosis of sciatica. Where would your patient complain of pain?

The posterior leg or thigh.

❑❑ What is thyrotoxicosis, and what are its causes?

A hypermetabolic state that occurs secondary to excess circulating thyroid hormone caused by thyroid hormone overdose, thyroid hyperfunction, or thyroid inflammation.

❑❑ What are the clinical features of myxedema coma?

Hypothermia (75%) and coma.

❑❑ Inflammation of the endorcardium is described by what term?

Endocarditis.

❑❑ Which hormone is associated with regulating the amount of sodium in the body?

Aldosterone.

❑❑ Excessive fluids move into cells when the secretion of what hormone decreases?

ADH.

❑❑ What effect does propranolol have on blood sugar levels in diabetic patients?

Propranolol may precipitate hyperglycemia.

❑❑ What is the normal range of fasting blood sugar?

50-80.

❑❑ What are the neurologic signs and symptoms of hypoglycemia?

Paresthesias, cranial nerve palsies, transient hemiplegia, diplopia, decerebrate posturing, and clonus.

❑❑ What are the signs and symptoms of thyroid storm?

Tachycardia, fever, diaphoresis, increased CNS activity, heart failure, coma, and death.

❑❑ What is the prognosis for a patient with amyotrophic lateral sclerosis (ALS)?

Approximately 10 years of life after the onset of symptoms. ALS, also known as Lou Gehrig's disease, involves the progressive loss of the anterior horn cell function of the motor neurons. No sensory abnormalities are involved, just muscular atrophy and gradual weakness.

❑❑ Cardiac isoenzymes are specific to heart muscle tissues and are useful in diagnosing what cardiac diseases?

Acute myocardial infarction.

❏❏ What are some of the purposes of cardiac catherization?

Measurement of the pressure in the heart chambers and pulmonary arteries. Obtainment of blood samples from the heart. Detection of congenital or acquired defects.

❏❏ What is the common term for arterial spasms resulting in a decreased flow of blood through the coronary arteries?

Angina pectoris.

❏❏ What occurs when one of the coronary arteries or its branches becomes suddenly occluded?

Myocardial infection.

❏❏ What is the legal definition of blindness?

Visual acuity of 20/400, or worse.

❏❏ Name some of the causes of cerebral palsy.

70% of all cases are idiopathic. Other causes include inutero infections, chromosomal abnormalities, or strokes. Cerebral palsy is a defect in the central nervous system that occurs prenatally, perinatally, or before the age of 3. Mental retardation occurs in 25% of patients with cerebral palsy.

❏❏ Differentiate between decerebrate and decorticate posturing.

Decerebrate: Elbows and legs are extended which is indicative of a midbrain lesion.
Decorticate: Elbows are flexed, legs are extended. This suggests a lesion in the thalamic region.

❏❏ A patient opens his eyes to voice, makes incomprehensible sounds, and withdraws to painful stimulus. What is his GCS?

9.

❏❏ Define the properties of the Glasgow Coma Scale.

Eye opening	Verbal activity	Motor activity
4. Spontaneous	5. Oriented	6. Obeys command
3. To command	4. Confused	5. Localizes pain
2. To pain	3. Inappropriate	4. Withdraws to pain
1. None	2. Incomprehensible	3. Flexion to pain
	1. None	2. Extension to pain
		1. None

❏❏ Differentiate between partial and generalized seizures.

Partial seizures arise from a single focus and may spread out, whereas generalized seizures involve the whole cerebral cortex. Absence and grand mal seizures are examples of generalized seizures. Generalized and complex partial seizures involve a loss of consciousness.

❏❏ Recurrent seizures in patients with a history of febrile seizures generally occur in what time

frame?

About 85% occur within the first 2 years. The younger the child, the more likely recurrence will happen. If a patient has a febrile seizure in the first year of life, the recurrence rate is 50%. If it occurs in the second year, the recurrence is only 25%.

❑❑ **What are the chances that a child will develop Huntington's chorea if her father has the same disease?**

50%.

❑❑ **What is the most common presenting symptom of MS?**

Optic neuritis (about 25%).

❑❑ **A 32-year-old female complains of periods of weakness, especially when she chews her food. She presents with ptosis, diplopia, and dysarthria. Her muscles weaken with repetitive exercise. What is the most probable diagnosis?**

Myasthenia Gravis. A patient with myasthenia gravis produces autoimmune antibodies against her own acetylcholine receptors in the neuromuscular junction. Therefore, giving exogenous anticholinesterase will lead to an increase of acetylcholine and thereby relieve the symptoms.

❑❑ **A resting tremor is most likely related to what disease?**

Parkinson disease. The tremors of Parkinson disease are generally asymmetrical and have the characteristic "pill rolling" appearance. The brain lesion is located in the substantia nigra.

❑❑ **Your male patient has a diagnosis of emphocele. Define emphocele.**

A collection of pus in a sacculated cavity such as the scrotum.

❑❑ **APAP (acetaminophen) poisoning can produce damage to which internal organ?**

The liver.

❑❑ **Define othopneic.**

When the patient is unable to breathe except in a sitting position.

❑❑ **What antihypertensive agent may induce cyanide poisoning?**

Nitroprusside. One molecule of sodium nitroprusside contains 5 molecules of cyanide. In order to prevent toxicity, sodium thiosulfate should be infused with sodium nitroprusside at a ratio of 10:1, thiosulfate to nitroprusside.

❑❑ **Why is the venous blood of the patient with cyanide poisoning described as being "cherry red"?**

In cyanide poisoning, electron transport is inhibited leading to an inability to utilize oxygen as an electron acceptor. Therefore, venous blood will contain a high partial pressure of oxygen.

❏❏ **What are the signs and symptoms of phenytoin toxicity?**
Seizure, heart blocks, bradyarrhythmias, hypotension, and coma. All dangerous cardiovascular complications of phenytoin overdose result from parenteral administration. High levels after PO doses do not cause such signs in a stable patient.

❏❏ **Describe the pathophysiologic features of HIV.**

HIV attacks the T4 helper cells. The genetic material of HIV consists of singlestranded RNA. HIV has been found in semen, vaginal secretions, blood and blood products, saliva, urine, cerebrospinal fluid, tears, alveolar fluid, synovial fluid, breast milk, transplanted tissue, and amniotic fluid. There has not been documentation of infection from casual contact.

❏❏ **How quickly do patients infected with HIV become symptomatic?**

The mean incubation time is about 8.23 years for adults and 1.97 years for children less than 5 years old. Between 5-10% of HIV patients develop symptoms within 3 years of seroconversion. Predictive characteristics include a low T4 count and a hematocrit less than 40.

❏❏ **Name the most common causes of fever in HIV-infected patients.**

HIV related fever, Mycobacterium aviumintracellular, CMV, and non-Hodgkin's and Hodgkin's lymphoma.

❏❏ **What is the most common cause of focal encephalitis in AIDS patients?**

Toxoplasmosis. Symptoms include focal neurologic deficits, headache, fever, altered mental status, and seizures. Ring-enhancing lesions are evident on CT.

❏❏ **What is the most common opportunistic infection in AIDS patients?**

PCP. Symptoms may include a nonproductive cough and dyspnea. A chest x-ray may reveal diffuse interstitial infiltrates or it may be negative.

❏❏ **What is the most common gastrointestinal complaint in AIDS patients?**

Diarrhea. Hepatomegaly and hepatitis are also typical. Cryptosporidium and Isospora are common causes of prolonged watery diarrhea.

❏❏ **What is the risk of contracting HIV infection after an occupational exposure?**

0.32% for needle sticks and 0.08% for mucus membrane exposure to high risk body fluids. Approximately 80% of the occupational exposure-related infections are from needle sticks.

❏❏ **Define homeostasis.**

The equilibrium of chemical and physical properties of body fluids.

❏❏ **How should a rabies wound be treated?**

Wound care of a suspected rabies bite should include debridement and irrigation. The physician will not suture the wound, it should remain open. This will decrease the rabies infection by 90%.

❐❐ **When are patients most likely to acquire Lyme disease?**
Late spring to late summer, with the highest incidence in July.

❐❐ **What is the most common site of herpes simplex I virus infection?**

The lower lip. First the lip itches and burns, then the small vesicle with the red base appears. These lesions are painful and can frequently recur since the virus remains in the sensory ganglia. Stress, sun, and illness generally trigger recurrences.

❐❐ **You are doing a rotation on the burn unit and on orientation you are told the "rule of nines system" is used. What does this term mean?**

The Rule of Nines formula is used to estimate the amount of body surface covered by burns.

❐❐ **What are the 3 main types of urinary incontinence?**

Stress, urge, and overflow.

❐❐ **T/F: What drug may be injected into the bursae in acute bursitis.**

Hydrocortisone.

❐❐ **T/F: Allergy is an abnormal response of the immune system caused by any substance to which an individual is hypersensitive.**

True.

❐❐ **What are the most common food allergies?**

Dairy products, eggs, and nuts.

❐❐ **When do the clinical manifestations of a drug allergy usually become apparent?**

1-2 weeks after starting the drug.

❐❐ **Which drug most commonly causes true allergic reactions?**

Penicillin, which accounts for approximately 90% of all true allergic reactions. 95% of fatal anaphylactic reactions are caused by penicillin. Parenterally administered penicillin is more than twice as likely to cause a fatal anaphylactic reaction than the orally administered type.

❐❐ **How long after exposure to an allergen does anaphylaxis occur?**

Between 1 second and one hour of exposure.

❐❐ **Anaphylaxis-related deaths are primarily caused by penicillin. What is the second most common cause?**

Insect stings. Approximately 100 deaths in the U.S. occur annually because of anaphylaxis that is induced by insect stings.

❒❒ A patient presents with fever, acute polyarthritis, and migratory arthritis a few weeks after a bout of Streptococcal pharyngitis. What disease should be suspected?

Acute rheumatic fever. Although the early symptoms may be nonspecific, a physical exam eventually reveals signs of arthritis (60-75%), carditis (30%), choreiform movements (10%), erythema marginatum, or subcutaneous nodules.

❒❒ What treatment should be started after the diagnosis of acute rheumatic fever has been made?

Penicillin or erythromycin should be given even if cultures for Group A Streptococcus are negative. High dose aspirin therapy is used at an initial dose of 75-100 mg/kg/day. Carditis or congestive heart failure is treated with prednisone, 1-2 mg/kg/day.

❒❒ Immobilization of a patient may result in what type of infection?

Hypostatic pneumonia.

❒❒ What is the treatment of choice for patients in anaphylactic shock?

Epinephrine, 0.3-0.5 mg intravenously. If there is no IV access, inject the medication into the venous plexus at the base of the tongue.

❒❒ How long should a patient with a generalized anaphylactic reaction be observed?

For at least 24 hours.

❒❒ A patient who is on chronic steroids presents with weakness, depression, fatigue, and postural dizziness. What pathological process should be suspected? What is the treatment?

Adrenal insufficiency. The treatment is to administer large "stress doses" of steroids.

❒❒ What is Legg-Calvé-Perthes disease, how does it present, and who is affected?

Legg-Calvé-Perthes disease is avascular necrosis of the femoral head, presenting in children who are between the ages of 2-13 years. Symptoms include subacute groin, hip, and knee pain that worsens with activity. This disease is also known as Coxa Plana.

❒❒ What is the most important abnormality of renal function when the level of potassium is low in the body?

The inability of the kidneys to concentrate urine.

❒❒ What are the most common causes of allergic contact dermatitis?

Poison oak, poison ivy, and poison sumac. They are responsible for more cases of contact dermatitis than all the other allergens combined.

❒❒ Why does scratching spread poison oak and ivy?

The antigenic resin contaminates the hands and fingernails, and is thereby spread by rubbing or scratching. A single contaminated finger can produce more than 500 reactive groups of lesions.

❑❑ **How is the antigen of poison oak or poison ivy inactivated?**

Careful washing with soap and water destroys the antigen. Special attention must be paid to the fingernails, otherwise the antigenic resin can be carried for weeks.

❑❑ **What rheumatologic ailment can produce valvular heart disease?**

Rheumatic fever.

❑❑ **What is the most common cause of acute renal failure?**

Acute tubular necrosis. Acute tubular necrosis occurs after a toxic or an ischemic injury to the kidneys caused from shock, surgery, or rhabdomyolysis.

❑❑ **What occurs when the heart fails to pump an adequate amount of blood to vital organs?**

Cardiogenic shock.

❑❑ **This acute condition is caused by cardiac failure, but the pulmonary system is affected.**

Acute pulmonary edema.

❑❑ **Which vascular system is affected by CHF?**

Pulmonary vascular system.

❑❑ **How does the pain associated with epididymitis differ from that produced by prostatitis?**

Epididymitis: The pain begins in the scrotum or groin and radiates along the spermatic cord. It intensifies rapidly, is associated with dysuria, and is relieved with scrotal elevation (Prehn's sign).
Prostatitis: Patients will have frequency, dysuria, urgency, bladder outlet obstruction, and retention. They may have low back pain and perineal pain associated with fever, chills, arthralgias, and myalgias.

❑❑ **What are some causes of false-positive hematuria?**

Food coloring, beets, paprika, rifampin, phenothiazines, Dilantin, myoglobin, or menstruation.

❑❑ **What 4 clinical findings indicate acute glomerulonephritis (GN)?**

Oliguria, hypertension, pulmonary edema, and urine sediment containing red blood cells, white blood cells, protein, and red blood cell casts.

❑❑ **What is the most common cause of hematuria?**

Lesions of the bladder or lower urinary tract. When hematuria originates in a kidney, the probable causes are polycystic kidney disease and nephropathy.

❑❑ **What is the 5-year recurrence rate for kidney stones?**

50%. The 10-year recurrence rate is 70%.

❏❏ **What percentage of patients spontaneously pass kidney stones?**

80%. This is largely dependent on size. 75% of stones less than 4 mm pass spontaneously, while only 10% of those larger than 6 mm pass spontaneously. Analgesics and increased fluid intake aid in outpatient management of kidney stones.

❏❏ **What is the post void residual volume that suggests urinary retention?**

A volume greater than 60 cc.

❏❏ **What is the most common cause of nephrotic syndrome in adults?**

Idiopathic glomerulonephritis.

❏❏ **What is the definition of oliguria?**

A urine output of less than 500 mL/day.

❏❏ **What is the definition of anuria?**

Urine output of less than 100 mL/day.

❏❏ **What is the most common origin of proteinuria?**

Pathology of the glomerulus. Other origins are tubular pathology or over production of protein.

❏❏ **What are the risk factors for pyelonephritis?**

Multiple prior UTI's, longer duration of symptoms, recent pyelonephritis, diabetes, and anatomic abnormalities. Immunocompromised patients and indigents are also at greater risk.

❏❏ **What is the most common cause of chronic renal failure?**

NIDDM.

❏❏ **When are the symptoms related to renal insufficiency displayed?**

When 90% of the nephrons have been destroyed. Hypertension, diabetes mellitus, glomerulonephritis, polycystic kidney disease, tubulointerstitial disease, and obstructive uropathy are all causes of chronic renal failure.

❏❏ **What is the most common cause of intrinsic renal failure?**

Acute tubular necrosis (80-90%), resulting from either an ischemic injury or a nephrotoxic agent. Less frequent causes of intrinsic renal failure (10-20%) include vasculitis, malignant hypertension, acute GN, or allergic interstitial nephritis.

❏❏ **What is the life expectancy of chronic renal patients after the disease has progressed to the point of dialysis?**

If the patient is younger than 60, there is a 4-5-year survival. If he/she is over 60, life expectancy drops to just 2-3 years.

❑❑ **A slight increase or decrease in the concentration of what ion will cause the heart to stop?**

Potassium.

❑❑ **T/F: A bland diet would include chocolate.**

False.

❑❑ **Testicular torsion is most common in which age group?**

14-year-olds. Two-thirds of the cases occur in the second decade. The next most common group is newborns.

❑❑ **T/F: Testicular torsion frequently follows a history of strenuous physical activity or occurs during sleep.**

True.

❑❑ **What is the definitive treatment for testicular torsion?**

Bilateral orchiopexy in which the testes are surgically attached to the scrotum.

❑❑ **What is the most common cause of urethritis in males?**

Neisseria gonorrhea, gonococcal urethritis, Chlamydia trachomatis, and nongonococcal urethritis.

❑❑ **What is the first-line of treatment for ventricular fibrillation in a hypothermic patient?**

Bretylium, NOT lidocaine.

❑❑ **A 14-year-old football player presents with light-headedness, headache, nausea, and vomiting. On exam, the patient has a HR of 110, RR 22, BP of 90/60, and is afebrile. Profuse sweating is noted. What is your diagnosis?**

Heat exhaustion. Treat with .9 NS IV fluid.

❑❑ **A 17-year-old marathon runner presents confused and combative. Temperature is 105°C. Why must renal function be monitored?**

The patient has heatstroke. Rhabdomyolysis may occur 2-3 days post injury. Recall that in heatstroke, volume depletion and dehydration may not always occur.

❑❑ **Treatment of heatstroke?**

Cool sponging, ice packs to groin and axilla, fanning, and iced gastric lavage. Antipyretics are not useful.

❑❑ **How should a honeybee's stinger be removed?**

Scrape it out. Squeezing with a tweezers or finger may increase envenomation.

❐❐ A 16-year-old presents with intense itching of the penis and the web spaces of his hands. What is your diagnosis?

Scabies frequently attacks the web spaces of the hands and feet. Small vesicles and papules may be present.

❐❐ Hypothermia is defined as a core temperature below what?

35°C.

❐❐ Heat loss can occur via radiation, convection, conduction, and evaporation. Which of these accounts for the greatest loss?

Radiation, followed by convection when not perspiring. If immersed, conduction causes the greatest heat loss.

❐❐ What are some of the nursing interventions for your patient receiving sealed internal radiation therapy?

Check vital signs frequently.
Encourage high fluid intake.
Check position of application every 4 hours.
Have call light and phone in easy reach.
Attach radiation symbol to door.
Follow precautions as ordered.
Observe for signs and symptoms of radiation reaction.
Maintain self-protection measures.

❐❐ Which types of blood loss are indicative of a bleeding disorder?

Spontaneous bleeding from many sites, bleeding from non-traumatic sites, delayed bleeding several hours after trauma, and bleeding into deep tissues or joints.

❐❐ Below what platelet count is spontaneous hemorrhage likely to occur?

< 10,000/mm3.

❐❐ How can an overdose of warfarin be treated? What are the advantages and disadvantages of each treatment?

Treatment depends on the severity of symptoms, not the degree of prolongation of the prothrombin time (PT). If there are no signs of bleeding, temporary discontinuation may be all that is necessary; if bleeding is present, treatment can be initiated with fresh frozen plasma (FFP) or Vitamin K.

Advantages of FFP: rapid repletion of coagulation factors and control of hemorrhage. Disadvantages: volume overload, possible viral transmission

Advantages of Vitamin K: ease of administration. Disadvantages: possible anaphylaxis when given IV; delayed onset of 12-24 hours; effects may last up to 2 weeks, making anticoagulation of the patient difficult or impossible.

❑❑ **What are the clinical complications of DIC?**

Bleeding, thrombosis, and purpura fulminans.

❑❑ **What 3 laboratory studies would be most helpful in establishing the diagnosis of DIC?**

1) Prothrombin time—prolonged.
2) Platelet count—usually low.
3) Fibrinogen level—low.

❑❑ **What are the most common hemostatic abnormalities in patients infected with HIV?**

Thrombocytopenia and acquired circulating anticoagulants (causes prolongation of the PTT).

❑❑ **What is the leading cause of death in hemophiliacs?**

AIDS.

❑❑ **What types of clinical crises are seen in patients with sickle-cell disease?**

Vaso-occlusive (thrombotic), hematologic (sequestration and aplastic), and infectious.

❑❑ **What are the mainstays of therapy for a patient in sickle-cell crisis?**

1) Hydration.
2) Analgesia.
3) Oxygen (only beneficial if patient is hypoxic).
4) Cardiac monitoring (if patient has history of cardiac disease or is having chest pain).

❑❑ **What are the 3 conditions under which the transfusion of PRBC's should be considered?**

1) Acute hemorrhage (blood loss > 1,500 ml).
2) Surgical blood loss > 2 L.
3) Chronic anemia (Hgb < 7–8 g/dL, symptomatic, or with underlying cardiopulmonary disease).

❑❑ **What factors indicate the need for typing and cross-matching of blood in an emergency setting?**

1) Evidence of shock from whatever cause.
2) Known blood loss > 1,000 ml.
3) Gross GI bleeding.
4) Hgb < 10; Hct < 30.
5) Potential of going to surgery with further significant blood loss.

❑❑ **What is the first step in treating all immediate transfusion reactions?**

Stop the transfusion.

❑❑ **What infection carries the highest risk of transmission by blood transfusion?**

Hepatitis C.

❑❑ **What is the currently approved emergency replacement therapy for massive hemorrhage?**

Type-specific, uncrossmatched blood (available in 10-15 minutes). Type O negative, whereas immediately life-saving in certain situations, carries the risk of life-threatening transfusion reactions.

❑❑ **What is the only crystalloid fluid compatible with packed RBC's?**

Normal saline.

❑❑ **What is the most common malignancy of the skin?**

Basal cell carcinoma. 80–90% of these lesions are found on the head and neck. Basal cell carcinoma appears as a pearly telangectasia with a central ulceration. These may spread locally, but they rarely metastasize.

❑❑ **Candida albicans infections of the skin are most commonly located where?**

In the intertriginous areas (i.e., in the folds of the skin, axilla, groin, under the breasts, etc.) Candida albicans appears as a beefy red rash with satellite lesions.

❑❑ **What is a carbuncle?**

A deep abscess that interconnects and extends into the subcutaneous tissue. Commonly seen in patients with diabetes, folliculitis, steroid use, obesity, heavy perspiration, and in areas of friction.

❑❑ **A mother brings her 14-year-old boy to you a week after a physician prescribed ampicillin for his pharyngitis. Mom says he developed a rash over his torso, arms, legs, and even the palms of his hands. On examination the patient has a rash in the places described. What might the child have other than pharyngitis?**

Infectious mononucleosis. In almost 95% of patients with Epstein Barr viruses that are treated with ampicillin, a rash will develop. The rash and subsequent desquamation will last about a week.

❑❑ **What is a furuncle?**

A deep, inflammatory nodule that grows out of superficial folliculitis.

❑❑ **What population has the highest incidence of melanoma?**

30–50-year-olds.

❑❑ **A black-and-blue spot is the result of injury to soft tissue. What is this called?**

Contusion.

❑❑ **What is the correct term for a broken bone with bone showing through the skin?**

Compound fracture.

❑❑ **What is a pilonidal abscess?**

An abscess which occurs in the gluteal fold as a result of disruption of the epithelial surface.

❒❒ **Where does a perirectal abscess originate?**

Anal crypts and burrows through the ischiorectal space. They may be perianal, perirectal, supralevator, or ischiorectal. Perianal abscesses which involve the supralevator muscle, ischiorectal space, or rectum require operative drainage.

❒❒ **What is the difference between viral and bacterial pneumonia on X-ray?**

Viral pneumonia appears as a patchy distribution throughout a lung. Bacterial pneumonia may affect one or more lobes of the lungs.

❒❒ **What is the difference between a lobectomy and pneumonectomy?**

A lobectomy involves the removal of a lobe (usually lower) of a lung, while a pneumonectomy is the removal of an entire lung.

❒❒ **A 17-year-old female has a rash over her elbows and her knees. On examination, you find that she has several plaques covered with silvery scales, which can be removed by scraping. These lesions are found only in the bodily areas previously mentioned. Examination of her nails reveals pitting in the nail beds. What is her probable prognosis?**

Psoriasis is an intermittent disease that may spontaneously disappear or may be life long. There may be associated arthritis in the distal interphalangeal joints; otherwise, the disease is limited to the skin and nails. Treatment is with hydration of the skin and topical mid-potency steroids.

❒❒ **A 60-year-old patient presents to your office complaining of greasy, red, scaly, plaques in her eyebrows, eyelids and nose that are spreading to the naso-labial folds. What patient population is this disease more likely to occur in?**

The above patient has seborrheic dermatitis. This can occur in anyone but is also a common problem in patients with HIV and Parkinson's disease. The infant form of the disease is "cradle cap."

❒❒ **A 72-year-old female comes to your office complaining of a painful red rash with crops of blisters on erythematous bases in a band-like distribution on the right side of her lower back spreading down and out towards her hip. What is the probable diagnosis?**

Shingles or herpes zoster disease. This is due to a reactivation of the dormant varicella virus in the sensory root ganglia of a patient with a history of chicken pox. The rash is in the distribution of the dermatome, in this case L5. It is most common in the elderly population or in patients who are immunocompromised. Treatment is with acyclovir and oral analgesics. This will help decrease the post herpetic neuralgia that is frequently associated with the disease.

❒❒ **Where is the most common site of eruption of herpes zoster?**

The thorax. Unlike chicken pox, shingles can recur.

❒❒ **What are the 2 phases of shingles?**

Eruptive and posterpetic.

❒❒ **Tinea capitis is most commonly seen in what age group?**

Children aged 4–14. This is a fungal infection of the scalp that begins as a papule around one hair shaft and then spreads to other follicles. The infection can cause the hairs to break off, leaving little black dot stumps and patches of alopecia. Trichophyton tonsurans is responsible for 90% of the cases. Wood's lamp examination will fluoresce only Microsporum infections, which are responsible for the remaining 10%. This is also called "ringworm of the scalp."

❑❑ What are the 3 most common causes of acute urticaria?

1) Medicine.
2) Arthropod bites.
3) Infection.

Urticaria, also known as hives or wheels, is a localized swelling, which is due to a cytokine mediated increase in vascular permeability.

❑❑ What is the most common location of verrucae vulgaris?

This is the common wart. It is usually located on the back of the hands or fingers and is caused by HPV.

❑❑ What can be done to prevent the development of decubitus ulcers?

Frequently change the patients position (q 2 hours), keep the skin dry and clean, use protective padding at potential sites of ulceration (i.e., heel pads or ankle pads), and keep patients on "egg-crate" mattresses or the like. In diabetics, encourage daily foot examination.

❑❑ According to the 1990 census, what percentage of Americans are over 65?

12 .6%.

❑❑ How many stages are associated with pressure ulcers?

4.

❑❑ T/F: Stage 2 pressure ulcers involve both the dermis and the epedermis.

True.

❑❑ Describe each pressure sore stage.

Stage 1: Inflammatory response with or without a break in the skin.
Stage 2: Shallow ulcer with distant edges and drainage surrounded by an area of redness, heat and swelling. The dermis is involved.
Stage 3: Irregular ulceration involving subcutaneous fat. Drainage may be copious.
Stage 4: Deep ulceration that extends into the muscle with visualization of ligaments and bone. The wound and drainage are foul smelling and the edges are thick and pigmented.

❑❑ How do the sleep patterns of the elderly differ from those of younger age groups?

The elderly spend less time asleep; they have an increased number of nocturnal awakenings and decreased REM. Also, they fall asleep earlier and wake up earlier than their younger counterparts.

❑❑ **The administration of aminoglycoside or cephalosporins to an elderly patient who is dehydrated may cause what?**

Acute renal failure secondary to tubulointerstitial injury. This may also occur if the above mentioned drugs are given to elderly patients on furosemide or with preexisting renal disease.

❑❑ **What are the 4 ways cancers can be treated?**

Surgery, chemotherapy, radiotherapy, and biotherapy.

❑❑ **T/F: Although both normal and abnormal cells are affected by radiation, malignant cells are more susceptible to ionizing rays than normal cells.**

True.

❑❑ **A doctor has written an order that you cannot understand. What should you do?**

Ask your team leader or charge nurse to try to interpret or call the doctor and confirm the order.

❑❑ **What is the sundown syndrome in the elderly?**

Hallucinations and delusions that occur at night time.

❑❑ **What is the most common cause of obstruction in the large bowel in the elderly?**

Fecal impaction. Other causes are stenosing diverticula, neoplasms, and volvulus colon. Adhesions are rarely a cause of obstruction in the large bowel.

❑❑ **What skin problem do the elderly most commonly seek medical attention for?**

Pruritus.

❑❑ **The most common causes of dysphagia in the elderly population include:**

Hiatal hernia, reflux esophagitis, webs/rings, and cancer.

❑❑ **What is the major nursing consideration for a patient who has received pre-operative medication?**

Safety of the patient.

❑❑ **You are to transport your patient to the surgical unit this morning. What are some to the nursing considerations to be aware of?**

Safety.
Comfort.
All records should accompany patient.
Patency of the IV, if ordered.
Pre-operative medications given.
All consents should be signed before pre-operative medication is given.
Inform family members of the appropriate waiting area.

❒❒ **What is the most common cause of cataract development?**

Old age. Cataracts can occur congenitally from medication or trauma. Slit lamp examination may show absent red reflex and a gray clouding of the lens.

❒❒ **What is the most common cause of blindness in the elderly?**

Senile macular degeneration. Such patients have a gradual loss of central vision. The macule appears hemorrhagic or pigmented. This is due to atrophic degeneration of the retinal vessels that results in leaking vessels, fibrosis, and scarring of the retina.

❒❒ **What is the most common non-traumatic cause of dementia?**

Alzheimer's disease. At 65, 10% of the population has Alzheimer's; by 85, the percentage increases to half. Multi-infarct dementia is the second most common cause of non-traumatic dementia.

❒❒ **What is the first symptom of Alzheimer's disease?**

Progressive memory loss. This is followed by disorientation, personality changes, language difficulty, and other symptoms of dementia.

❒❒ **What is the prognosis for patients with Alzheimer's disease?**

This is an irreversible disease. Death occurs 5–10 years after presumptive diagnosis.

❒❒ **Differentiate between dementia and delirium.**

Dementia - Irreversible impaired functioning secondary to changes/deficits in memory, spatial concepts, personality, cognition, language, motor and sensory skills, judgment, or behavior. There is no change in consciousness.

Delirium - A reversible organic mental syndrome reflecting deficits in attention, organized thinking, orientation, speech, memory, and perception. Patients are frequently confused, anxious, excited, and have hallucinations. A change in consciousness can be observed.

❒❒ **When is a post void residual urine considered abnormal?**

When it exceeds 200 mL.

❒❒ **What is the most common complication of a pressure ulcer?**

Sepsis.

❒❒ **What vitamin is effective in treating pressure ulcers?**

Vitamin C.

❒❒ **What are the major clinical findings in Alzheimer's patients?**

Memory loss, delusions, hallucinations, language impairment, loss of visual and spatial orientation, and loss of interest in life activities.

❑❑ **What agent is best used for cleaning an infected pressure ulcer?**

Saline.

❑❑ **What bacteria is the most common cause of UTI's in uncatheterized elderly patients?**

E. coli.

❑❑ **In the elderly, what is a common side effect of verapamil?**

Constipation.

❑❑ **Parkinson-like side effects are common with which class of drugs?**

Neuroleptics. Parkinson-like side effects can be seen with perphenazine (Trilafon), chlorpromazine (Thorazine), reserpine, haloperidol (Haldol), metoclopramide (Reglan), and the illicit meperidine (Demerol) analog MPTP.

❑❑ **In the elderly, what is the most common cause of death due to infection in the community, in institutions, and in the hospital?**

In the community and institutions, it is bacterial pneumonia; and in hospitals, it is UTI's.

❑❑ **T/F: Candida species and Escherichia coli are common organisms found to be the cause of endogenous UTIs.**

True.

❑❑ **What is the most common cause of drug-induced hallucinations in the geriatric population?**

Propranolol.

❑❑ **Why is it unsafe to place a geriatric patient on digoxin and Lasix?**

Hypokalemia and digoxin toxicity may result.

❑❑ **An acute state of confusion is also known as what?**

Delirium. Diagnostic features include reduced level of consciousness, disorganized sleep-wake cycles, disturbances in attention, global cognitive impairment, and decreased or increased psychomotor activity.

❑❑ **What is the most common cause of abdominal pain in the elderly?**

Constipation.

❑❑ **What is the most commonly found risk factor in patients diagnosed with Alzheimer's disease?**

Family history of dementia.

❑❑ What is the major risk of tricyclic antidepressants in the elderly?

Orthostatic hypotension which leads to falls.

❑❑ What is the most common source of sepsis in the elderly?

Respiratory > Urinary > Intra-abdominal.

❑❑ What is the most common mechanism of injury in the elderly?

Falls > MVA > Burns > Assaults.

❑❑ A 24-year-old male presents to the ED complaining of pleuritic pain, palpitations, dyspnea, dizziness, and tingling in his arms and legs. What is a possible cause or these symptoms if cardiac dysfunction is ruled out?

Hyperventilation syndrome. This is frequently associated with anxiety. The tingling is due to decreased carbonate in the blood.

❑❑ What are the American Cancer Society's 1996 recommendations for mammography?

Every 1–2 years after age 40. Annually after age 50.

❑❑ What are the risk factors for breast cancer, and how do they compare with the risk factors for endometrial cancer?

Risk factors for both cancers include nulliparity, early menarche, late menopause, significant amounts of unopposed estrogen, and prior ovarian, endometrial, or breast cancer. Unopposed estrogen is a much greater risk in endometrial cancer than in breast cancer. Risk factors specific to breast cancer include family history, age over 40, high fat intake, radiation of the breast, or cellular atypia in fibrocystic disease.

❑❑ What is the number one cause of UTI's?

E. coli. Other causative agents are also Gram-negative.

❑❑ What are the contraindications to administration of oral iodine or barium contrast?

Barium cannot be given when complete colon obstruction exists or intestinal perforation is suspected. Severe allergy to iodine is the only contraindication to oral iodine-containing preparations.

❑❑ The magnetic fields of a MRI can be detrimental to patients with what?

Ferrous metal in their body or electrical equipment whose function can be disrupted by strong magnetic fields. Examples include pacemakers, metal foreign bodies in the eye (welders, sheet metal workers, artists who work with metal, etc.), ferromagnetic cerebral aneurysm clips (unless they are made of nonmagnetic steel), and cochlear implants. Relative contraindications for a MRI include certain prosthetic heart valves, implantable defibrillators, bone growth, and neurostimulators. One might also include patients who are claustrophobic.

❑❑ Define a nuclear family.

A family that consists of a husband, wife, and children.

❑❑ T/F: A disinfectant is a bacterial solution.

True.

❑❑ What are the top 10 causes of death in the U.S.?

1) Heart disease	6) Pneumonia and Influenza
2) Cancer	7) Diabetes
3) Stroke	8) HIV
4) COPD	9) Suicide
5) Accidents	10) Homicide

❑❑ Does a nonsmoker who has been married to a smoker for 25 years have a greater risk of lung cancer than a nonsmoker who has not lived with a smoker?

Yes. The risk is 1.34 times as greater than that of a person living in a smoke-free environment.

❑❑ What percentage of lung cancer is related to smoking?

80%.

❑❑ What cancer causes the most deaths in men?

Lung cancer > prostate cancer > colorectal cancer.

❑❑ What is the biggest risk factor for prostate cancer?

Age. The median age for diagnosis of prostate cancer is 72.

❑❑ Name 7 risk factors for malignant melanoma.

1) Fair skin
2) Sensitivity to sunlight
3) Excessive exposure to the sun
4) Dysplastic moles
5) 6 or more moles >.5 cm in diameter
6) Prior basal or squamous cell carcinoma
7) Parental history of skin cancer

Basal and squamous cell carcinomas are slow growing tumors that rarely metastasize.

❑❑ What percentage of melanomas occur in sun–exposed areas?

Only 65%! A good screen of all surface area is important. In African–American, Hispanic, and Asian patients, acral lentigines melanomas are more common. Careful examination of subungual, palmar, and plantar surfaces is important in these populations.

❑❑ Which malignancies are more common in obese individuals?

Endometrial cancer, breast cancer (postmenopausal), gallbladder cancer, biliary cancer, prostate cancer, and colorectal cancer.

❒❒ **Obesity is a risk factor for what common diseases?**

CAD, NIDDM, HTN, left ventricular hypertrophy, sleep apnea, cholelithiasis, pulmonary emboli, and osteoarthritis.

❒❒ **Before administering any medication to a client, what should you check?**

Drug allergies.

❒❒ **What immunizations do healthy senior citizens need?**

Tetanus booster every 10 years, influenza vaccination every year, and a pneumococcal vaccination.

❒❒ **What vaccines should be administered to adults?**

1) Hepatitis B vaccine (For patients at high risk—healthcare workers, homosexuals, and IV drug users)
2) Influenza vaccine (Should be given yearly to elderly patients or patients with chronic illness)
3) MR (Most often required by school institutions, it should be given to all patients without immunity)
4) Pneumococcal vaccine (Should be given once to patients over 65 or to any patient with a chronic illness)
5) Tetanus/diphtheria (A primary series and then booster every 10 years. All adults should receive this vaccine.)

❒❒ **A patient comes in for vaccinations and has a URI and a fever of 37.5°C. Can you administer vaccines to this patient?**

Yes. URI or gastrointestinal illness are not contraindications to vaccination. Fever may be as high as 38°C and the vaccine still administered. Likewise, use of antibiotics or recent exposure to illness is not a reason to delay vaccination.

❒❒ **A positive reaction to the Mantoux skin test in a person with HIV is how many mm?**

> 5 mm. In individuals with risk factors for TB, induration must be > 10 mm. For those with no risk factors, induration must be > 15 mm to be positive.

❒❒ **When should the influenza vaccine be given?**

In September or October, about 1–2 months before the influenza season begins. The vaccine, unlike amantadine, is protective against influenza A and B.

❒❒ **What is a contraindication to the administration of the influenza vaccine?**

A history of anaphylactic hypersensitivity to eggs or their products.

❒❒ **Are diabetic patients on oral hypoglycemics who mix their medication with alcohol more likely to become hyper or hypoglycemic?**

Hypoglycemic.

❑❑ **What is recommended in the prevention of hemorrhoids?**

Fiber supplements and stool softeners.

❑❑ **What is the diet recommended to reduce the risk of colon cancer?**

Decrease fat in the diet (especially saturated fat), increase fiber, increase cruciferous vegetables, decrease ETOH, and decrease smoked, salted, or nitrate-based foods.

❑❑ **What are the risk factors for colon cancer?**

Age over 50, familial polyposis (100%), ulcerative colitis, Crohn's disease, radiation exposure, benign adenomas, and previous history of colon cancer.

❑❑ **Name some drugs that when overdosed can lead to cardiac arrhythmias and death.**

Digoxin, antiarrhythmic drugs, cocaine, tricyclic antidepressants, darvon/darvocet, and phenothiazines.

❑❑ **What nutritional deficiencies may lead to apthous ulcers?**

B-12, folate, and iron deficiencies.

❑❑ **A 22-year-old healthy male who has no significant medical history and is taking no medication comes to your office complaining of a creamy white coat on his tongue. This substance easily rubs off, revealing an erythematous base. What should you be concerned about?**

HIV. In a patient who has no obvious reason for having an overgrowth of oral candida, HIV should be suspected. This patient does not have cancer, systemic illness, neutropenia, diabetes, adrenal insufficiency, nutritional deficiencies, or an immunocompromised state—all common causes for oral thrush overgrowth.

❑❑ **According to Holmes and Rahe, what are life's top 10 most stressful events? (Hint: taking the boards is not on the list.)**

1) Death of spouse or child
2) Divorce
3) Separation
4) Institutional detention
5) Death of close family member
6) Major personal injury or illness
7) Marriage
8) Job loss
9) Marital reconciliation
10) Retirement

❑❑ **Which organ is most commonly injured in a blunt trauma?**

The spleen. Generalized abdominal pain with radiation to the left shoulder subsequent to a blunt trauma indicates splenic rupture. Splenic rupture can also occur following infectious mononucleosis.

❑❑ **Which type of malignancy is most commonly associated with the AIDS disease?**

Kaposi's sarcoma with Non-Hodgkin's lymphoma coming in second.

❑❑ **Where are Kaposi's sarcoma lesions found?**

Everywhere—both inside and out. This type of lesion typically occurs on the face, neck, arms, back, thighs, and in the lungs, lymphatic system, and the GI system.

❒❒ **How many years does a patient usually have to live after being diagnosed with HIV?**

10 years. Most patients eventually die from PCP.

❒❒ **How is jaundice diagnosed in an African-American patient?**

Darkly pigmented patients often have subconjunctival fat that results in yellowing the sclera. In patients where icterus is suspected, it is imperative to examine the edges of the cornea and the posterior hard palate.

❒❒ **How does pallor appear in a black patient?**

The skin is yellow/brown or gray due to the loss of the underlying red tones. The conjunctiva will appear pale.

❒❒ **What is the most common cause of hypercalcemia?**

Hyperparathyroidism. This condition accounts for 60% of ambulatory hypercalcemics.

❒❒ **What is the most common cause of nongonococcal urethritis?**

Chlamydia trachomatis. Ureaplasma urealyticum is another common cause.

❒❒ **What is the most common cause of epididymitis?**

Chlamydia trachomatis.

❒❒ **Which strain of influenza is more common in adults and which strain is more common in children?**

Adults: Influenza A. Children: Influenza B.

❒❒ **What are some of the key features of Guillain-Barré syndrome?**

Guillain-Barré syndrome is a lower motor neuron disease which commonly affects people who are between the ages of 30 and 40. It presents as an ascending weakness involving the legs more than the arms. A sensory component may be present. Bulbar muscles are usually involved late in the course of the disease. Reflexes are affected early. Paralysis can progress rapidly; recovery is usually slow, but it is almost always complete.

❒❒ **What formula should be used to calculate the fluid requirements for resuscitation of a burn victim?**

2-4 mL/kg/% of total body surface area/day. One-half of this is given in the first 8 hours.

❒❒ **What animals are the most prevalent vectors of rabies in the world? In the U.S.?**

Worldwide, the dog is the most common carrier of rabies.
In the U.S., the skunk has become the most common carrier of disease. Bats, raccoons, cows, dogs, foxes and cats (in descending order) are also sources.

❑❑ **Describe the signs and symptoms of spinal shock.**

Spinal shock represents complete loss of spinal cord function below the level of injury. Patients have flaccid paralysis, complete sensory loss, areflexia, and loss of autonomic function. Such patients are usually bradycardic, hypotensive, hypothermic, and vasodilated.

❑❑ **The doctor orders a sputum C&S on your patient. What part of the exam is your responsibility?**

The collection of the sputum, if not specifically ordered by respiratory services.

❑❑ **What is the best time to instruct your patient on the collection of the sputum?**

In the morning, when sputum production is at its greatest.

❑❑ **What are the classic signs and symptoms of TB?**

Night sweats, fever, weight loss, malaise, cough, and a green/yellow sputum which most commonly is seen in the mornings.

❑❑ **What is the most common cause of paralytic ileus?**

Surgery.

❑❑ **What is the incubation period for hepatitis A?**

30 days. An RNA virus causes this disease.

❑❑ **How is hepatitis A transmitted?**

By the oral fecal route. No carrier state exists.

❑❑ **What type of hepatitis is caused by a DNA virus?**

Hepatitis B. The incubation period is 90 days.

❑❑ **How do steroids function in the treatment of asthma?**

Steroids increase cAMP, decrease inflammation, and aid in restoring the function of ß-adrenergic responsiveness to adrenergic drugs.

❑❑ **What is the most common cause of hyperthyroidism?**

Grave's disease (toxic diffuse goiter).

❑❑ **What is another name for life-threatening hypothyroidism?**

Myxedema coma. This condition occurs in elderly women during the winter months and is stimulated by infection and stress.

❑❑ **What is primary adrenal insufficiency?**

Addison's disease, that is, failure of the adrenal cortex.

❒❒ **What are the signs and symptoms of Addison's disease?**

Hyperpigmentation, hyperkalemia, alopecia, and ascending paralysis secondary to hyperkalemia. Lab findings in Addison's disease indicate hypoglycemia, hyponatremia, hyperkalemia, and azotemia.

❒❒ **What are the principal signs and symptoms in adrenal crisis?**

Abdominal pain, hypotension, and shock. The common cause of adrenal crisis is withdrawal of steroids. Treatment of adrenal crisis is the administration of hydrocortisone (Solu-Cortef), 100 mg IV bolus and 100 mg added to the first liter of D5 0.9 NS.

❒❒ **What key lab results are expected with SIADH?**

Low serum sodium levels and high urine sodium levels (i.e., > 30).

❒❒ **What are the common anticholinergic compounds?**

Atropine, tricyclic antidepressants, antihistamines, phenothiazines, antiparkinsonian drugs, belladonna alkaloids, and some Solanaceae plants (i.e., deadly nightshade and jimson weed).

❒❒ **Describe the symptoms and signs of myasthenia gravis.**

Weakness and fatigability with ptosis, diplopia, and blurred vision are the initial symptoms in 40–70% of the patients. Bulbar muscle weakness is also prevalent with dysarthria and dysphagia.

❒❒ **Describe the key features of Ménière's disease, also known as endolymphatic hydrops.**

Vertigo, hearing loss, and tinnitus are the hallmarks of Ménière's disease. Ménière's disease typically presents with the rapid onset of vertigo and nausea/vomiting that lasts from hours to 1 day. Nystagmus may be spontaneous during the critical stage. Tinnitus may be present and is louder during the attacks. Sensorineural hearing loss may be occur. There may also be an aura with a sensation of fullness in the ear during an attack. Symptoms are unilateral in over 90% of patients, and recurring attacks are typical.

❒❒ **What disease should be suspected in a patient with a 2 week history of lower limb weakness?**

Guillain-Barré usually causes an ascending weakness which begins in the lower extremities. Conversely, the weakness is descending with botulism poisoning. Cranial nerves are typically affected first with myasthenia gravis.

❒❒ **What is the treatment for Wernicke's encephalopathy?**

Thiamine IV.

❒❒ **What electrolyte abnormality is commonly associated with the transfusion of packed red blood cells?**

Hypocalcemia secondary to citrate toxicity. Citrate, when rapidly infused, binds ionized calcium and therefore decreases the calcium level. Hyperkalemia may also develop with rapidly packed red blood cell transfusion, especially if the patient is in renal failure or if the blood products are old.

❒❒ **What are the common symptoms and signs of hyperthyroidism?**

Symptoms include weight loss, palpitations, dyspnea, edema, chest pain, nervousness, weakness, tremor, psychosis, diarrhea, hyperdefecation, abdominal pain, myalgias, and disorientation. Signs such as fever, tachycardia, wide pulse pressure, CHF, shock, thyromegaly, tremor, weakness, liver tenderness, jaundice, stare, and hyperkinesis are evident. Mental status changes include somnolence, obtundation, coma, or psychosis. Pretibial myxedema may also be found—a true misnomer!

❒❒ **Which type of drugs would you suspect your patient to be on with a diagnosis of congestive heart failure?**

Diuretics and intropic agents (digitalis).

❒❒ **What are some of the nursing interventions for a patient with a diagnosis of CHF?**

Observe for signs and symptoms of hyperkalemia.
Weigh daily.
Place in a Fowlers position for optimum respiratory comfort.
Observe for signs of fluid overload.

❒❒ **During your respiratory assessment, you assess for resonance. What is this?**

Resonance is a normal sound. It is hollow, low pitched, non-musical, and loudest where the chest is thinnest.

❒❒ **How long should you listen when assessing the respiratory system?**

For several respiratory cycles.

❒❒ **Name the 4 adventitious breath sounds.**

Crackles, rhonchi, wheezes, and pleural friction rub.

❒❒ **What is another term for crackles?**

Rales.

❒❒ **What are the signs and symptoms of organic brain syndrome?**

Onset may occur at any age. Symptoms include visual hallucinations and perceptions of the unfamiliar as familiar. Signs include mental status changes (such as disorientation, clouded sensorium, asterixis, or mild clonus) and focal neurologic signs. Vital signs are often within normal limits.

❒❒ **What is a hyphema?**

Blood in the anterior chamber of the eye. Keep the head elevated in these patients.

❒❒ **Describe the symptoms and signs of varicella (chicken pox).**

The onset of varicella rash is 1–2 days after prodromal symptoms of slight malaise, anorexia, and fever. The rash begins on the trunk and scalp, appearing as faint macules which later become vesicles.

❑❑ **Your patient is receiving external radiation therapy. What are some of the nursing interventions?**

Give reassurance and support.
Ensure skin markings are not removed.
Observe for radiation reactions.
Encourage a high-caloric, high protein diet.
Encourage high fluid intake.

❑❑ **What are some of the acute side effects of external radiation therapy (ERT)?**

Nausea, vomiting, diarrhea, skin reactions, erytherma, fatigue, stomatitis, and pneumonitis.

❑❑ **T/F: Nurses caring for female patients with cervical cesium implants should stay 3 feet from the patients bedside and avoid spending more than 30 minutes in the room.**

True.

❑❑ **Signs of tension pneumothorax on a physical exam include what?**

Tachypnea, unilateral absent breath sounds, tachycardia, pallor, diaphoresis, cyanosis, tracheal deviation, hypotension, and neck vein distention.

❑❑ **Do local anesthetics freely cross the blood brain barrier?**

Yes. Most systemic toxic reactions to local anesthetics involve the CNS or cardiovascular system.

❑❑ **What electrolyte disorder is associated with hypercalcemia?**

Hypokalemia.

❑❑ **What complication may arise when citrate is present in stored blood?**

Citrate binds calcium which can induce hypocalcemia in a patient receiving the blood.

❑❑ **What is the universal donor blood?**

Type Rh negative blood, type O.

❑❑ **What are the common presentations of a transfusion reaction?**

Myalgia, dyspnea, fever associated with hypocalcemia, hemolysis, allergic reactions, hyperkalemia, citrate toxicity, hypothermia, coagulopathies, and altered hemoglobin function.

❑❑ **Define strabismus.**

Strabismus is defined as a lack of parallelism of the visual axis of the eyes.

Esotropias are medially deviated, exotropias are laterally deviated.

❑❑ **Which type of acid base disturbance initially occurs with a salicylate overdose?**

Respiratory alkalosis. Approximately 12 hours later, an anion gap metabolic acidosis or mixed acid base picture may occur.

❑❑ **The best method for transporting an amputated extremity is:**

Wrap the extremity in sterile gauze moistened with saline. Place it in a waterproof plastic bag. Immerse this in ice water.

❑❑ **What mechanism is responsible for the highest number of injuries in the elderly?**

Falls. Most falls are caused by tripping, but other medical origins underlying the initial fall should always be sought.

❑❑ **T/F: A bursa is a small sac containing fluid that lubricates certain areas.**

True.

❑❑ **What is the term for the disease in which there is a high level of uric acid in the blood?**

Gout.

❑❑ **What joint is most commonly affected with gout?**

The great toe MCP joint.

❑❑ **Describe the key features of the Rocky Mountain Spotted Fever (RMSF) rash.**

The rash has a sandpaper type texture and begins on the face, neck, chest, and abdomen. It then spreads to extremities. Patients may also have strawberry tongue.

❑❑ **What is the best treatment for an acute hemorrhagic overdose of Coumadin?**

Treat with fresh frozen plasma. Vitamin K IM will aid in preventing a subsequent hemorrhage.

❑❑ **What is the most common transfusion reaction?**

Febrile.

❑❑ **A patient has had 3 days of diarrhea, which was abrupt in onset. The patient reports slimy green, malodorous stools that contain blood. In addition, the patient is febrile. What is the most likely cause?**

Salmonella.

❑❑ **What drug will most rapidly decrease K+?**

Calcium chloride IV (1–3 minutes).

❑❑ **What is a potential side effect of the use of Kayexalate?**

Kayexalate exchanges sodium for K+. As a result, sodium overload and CHF may occur.

❒❒ **What metabolic conditions will potentiate the toxic cardiac effects of digoxin?**
Hypokalemia and hypercalcemia.

❒❒ **What is the initial treatment for hypercalcemia?**

Saline and furosemide.

❒❒ **What vital sign might be affected with hypermagnesemia?**

Hypermagnesemia causes hypotension because it relaxes vascular smooth muscle. Deep tendon reflexes may disappear.

❒❒ **How low does the platelet count drop before spontaneous bleeding occurs?**

Below 50,000/mm3 spontaneous bleeding may occur. CNS bleeds usually do not occur until counts drop below 10,000/mm3.

❒❒ **What effect will heparin or warfarin overdose have on the prothrombin time (PT) and the partial thromboplastin time (PTT)?**

When administered in excessive doses, both cause increases in PT and PTT.

❒❒ **What are the symptoms of an elevated PTT you should teach a patient undergoing heparin therapy at home to recognize?**

Bleeding gums, epistaxis, petechiae, and blood in urine or stool.

❒❒ **Antacids containing Magnesium may cause:**

Diarrhea.

❒❒ **Antacids containing Aluminum may cause:**

Constipation.

❒❒ **Is hepatitis A associated with jaundice?**

Typically not, as more than 50% of the population has serologic evidence for hepatitis and do not recall being symptomatic.

❒❒ **What are the most common symptoms of a PE?**

Chest Pain (88%) and dyspnea (84%).

❒❒ **What effect does furosemide have on calcium excretion?**

Furosemide causes increased calcium excretion in the urine.

❒❒ **An elderly patient presents with the complaint of seeing halos around lights. What diagnosis is suspected?**

Glaucoma. Another presenting complaint of glaucoma is blurred vision. Also, consider digitalis toxicity.

❑❑ **A trauma patient has a closed head injury with suspected elevated intracranial pressure. What treatments should you anticipate will be ordered?**

Paralyze the patient and hyperventilate, maintain hypovolemia (fluid restrict), elevate the head of the bed to 30 degrees after the C-spine has been cleared, and consider mannitol 500 ml of a 20% solution.

❑❑ **How should a patient with heat stroke be treated?**

Cool the patient with lukewarm water and fans, pack the axillae, neck, and groin with ice, give fluids cautiously as large boluses of fluids may precipitate pulmonary edema, and treat shivering with chlorpromazine (Thorazine) 25–50 mg IV.

❑❑ **What complications can result from heat stroke?**

Renal failure, rhabdomyolysis, DIC, and seizures. Remember that antipyretics won't help.

❑❑ **An elderly patient presents with altered mental status, history of IDDM, and is hypoglycemic. Core temperature is 32°C. What endocrinologic condition is likely?**

Myxedema coma. Other clues to look for are history of thyroid surgery, hypothyroidism, and use of antithyroid medications.

❑❑ **What findings mark the presentation of a patient with rapidly progressive glomerulonephritis?**

Hematuria (most common), edema (periorbital), HTN, ascites, pleural effusion, rales, and anuria.

❑❑ **What is phimosis?**

A condition in which the foreskin cannot be retracted posterior to the glands. The preliminary treatment is a dorsal slit.

❑❑ **What is paraphimosis?**

A condition in which the foreskin is retracted posterior to the glands and cannot be advanced over the glands.

❑❑ **What are causes of priapism?**

Prolonged sex, leukemia, sickle cell trait and disease, blood dyscrasias, pelvic hematoma or neoplasm, syphilis, urethritis, and drugs including phenothiazines, prazosin, tolbutamide, anticoagulants, and corticosteroids.

❑❑ **Describe the presentation of a patient with Gardnerella vaginitis.**

On physical exam, note a frothy, grayish-white, fishy smelling vaginal discharge.

❑❑ **What hypersensitivity skin rashes are noted with phenytoin use?**

Lupus-like and Stevens-Johnson syndrome.

❑❑ What symptoms are expected with a phenytoin level of > 20, > 30, and > 40 µg/ml?

> 20: lateral gaze nystagmus.
> 30: lateral gaze nystagmus plus increased vertical nystagmus with upward gaze.
> 40: lethargy, confusion, dysarthria, and psychosis.

❑❑ Describe the effects of salicylate poisoning on the central nervous system.

Lethargy, confusion, seizures, and respiratory arrest.

❑❑ What are the signs of salicylate poisoning?

Hyperventilation, hyperthermia, mental status change, nausea, vomiting, abdominal pain, dehydration, diaphoresis, ketonuria, metabolic acidosis, and respiratory alkalosis.

❑❑ In an MI, when do CK levels begin to rise, and when do they peak?

CK levels begin to rise at 6–8 hours; they peak at 24–30; and they stabilize at 48.

❑❑ In an MI, when does LDH begin to rise, and when does it peak?

LDH-I (from heart) begins to rise at 12–24 hours; it peaks at 48–96.

❑❑ Hepatic failure is commonly associated with what anticonvulsant?

Valproic acid.

❑❑ A patient presents with fever, neck pain, and trismus. Exam reveals pharyngeal edema with tonsil displacement and edema of the parotid area. What is the diagnosis?

Parapharyngeal abscess.

❑❑ Who should receive prophylaxis after exposure to Neisseria meningitidis?

People living with the patient or having close intimate contact.

❑❑ At about what core body temperature does shivering cease?

30–32° C.

❑❑ Describe the skin lesion seen in Lyme disease.

A large distinct circular skin lesion called erythema chronicum migrans. It is an annular erythematous lesion with central clearing.

❑❑ What are the most common complaints in a patient with carbon monoxide poisoning?

Headache, dizziness, weakness, and nausea.

❑❑ What makes the first heart sound?

Closure of the mitral valve and left ventricular contraction.

❑❑ **The second heart sound?**

Closure of the pulmonary and aortic valves.

❑❑ **What is a common pathological cause of an S3?**

Congestive heart failure.

❑❑ **Does furosemide affect preload or afterload?**

Furosemide decreases preload.

❑❑ **What is the shorter of the 2 common carotid arteries?**

The right common artery.

❑❑ **Define embolism.**

An obstruction of a blood vessel by a foreign substances or a blood clot.

❑❑ **A quadriplegic complains of a severe headache. What should you do?**

Check for signs of urinary retention. If a Foley catheter is present check to see if it is patent.

❑❑ **Why would you be concerned if a quadriplegic suddenly develops a severe headache?**

It is a symptom of autonomic dysreflexia. Bladder distention is one of the most common causes.

❑❑ **A client with glaucoma is given timolol (Timoptic) eye drops and she asks how long she will have to take them. What is your response?**

The eyedrops will have to be taken for the rest of her life.

❑❑ **An elderly client complains of constipation. What simple advice could you give the patient?**

Increase fiber, fluids, and exercise daily as long as this does not interfere with any other medical condition.

❑❑ **When are clients with active TB considered to be non-contagious?**

After producing 3 consecutive sputum specimens that are free of M. tuberculosis.

❑❑ **Following a diagnosis of active TB, the patient asks when he can return to work. How should you respond?**

As long as the patient is compliant with his medication, he will probably produce 3 negative sputum specimens within 2-3 weeks, at which time he may return to work.

❑❑ **When monitoring a client following a CVA, what changes in vital signs should be reported to**

the M.D. immediately?

Increased blood pressure, decreased pulse, and decreased respiratory rate.

❒❒ **What could the above changes in vital signs indicate?**

An increase in intercranial pressure.

❒❒ **A patient with a cast complains of itching underneath his cast and tries to reach it with a pencil. What can you do to increase the patient's comfort?**

Advise the M.D. and request an antihistamine.

❒❒ **Before any surgery that requires general anesthesia, what technique should you teach the patient that will help prevent a postoperative infection?**

Turn, cough, and deep breathing exercises will help prevent atelectasis.

❒❒ **What are some of the symptoms when excess fluid volume disturbs cerebral functions?**

Confusion, unusual behavior, loss of attention, and aphasia.

❒❒ **What is the first step the doctor may take in treating volume excess?**

Fluid restriction.

❒❒ **What vital signs can be taken that will help determine fluid volume deficit?**

Orthostatic blood pressure and pulse.

❒❒ **What should you be aware of when taking vital signs in a patient with an arteriovenous fistula?**

Do not take the blood pressure in the arm containing the fistula.

❒❒ **A nurse's aide refuses to go into an HIV positive client's room because she is afraid of contracting AIDS. How should you respond?**

Teach the aide how the HIV is transmitted and the concept of universal precautions.

❒❒ **What effect would you expect phenylephrine hydrochloride (Neosynephrine) drops to have on the eye?**

Mydriasis (pupil dilation).

❒❒ **You would expect intraocular pressure to be affected in what way by administering Neosynephrine eye drops?**

It would increase.

❒❒ **Your patient has a G-tube feeding ordered. What should you assess for before starting the feeding?**

Patentcy of the tube, bowel sounds, residual gastric contents, rate of flow, conformation of the product, and the last blood sugar, if ordered.

❑❑ **A patient with a positive TB skin test asks what that means. How should you respond?**

A positive skin test means that the patient has been exposed to tuberculosis. It does not mean the patient has the active disease. A chest x-ray and further examination will be needed to determine active TB.

❑❑ **A client in renal failure is prescribed polystyrene sulfonate (Kayexalate). What is the most likely reason for administering this drug?**

Elevated potassium levels.

❑❑ **You instruct a patient after a modified radical mastectomy to protect her arm on the affected side from injury or infection. Why?**

Following surgery, the patient will have an increased chance of infection in the affected extremity due to lymph node removal.

❑❑ **Following abdominal surgery, a patient coughs. You note that the suture line has opened and a segment of bowel has been exposed. What should you do?**

Immediately have the patient flex his knees, place sterile gauze over the wound soaked in sterile saline, and notify the physician immediately.

❑❑ **You note that a patient's WBC is below 1,000 mm3. What special interventions would be called for?**

Reverse isolation precautions to decrease any risk of opportunistic infection.

❑❑ **Following an adrenalectomy, how long do patients need to take replacement medication?**

For the remainder of their life.

❑❑ **Following several weeks of radiation therapy, a patient is concerned because she feels weak and tired all the time. How should you respond?**

These symptoms are a normal side effect of radiation therapy.

❑❑ **What are some of the symptoms of disequilibrium syndrome in a patient with chronic renal failure?**

Hypertension, headache, confusion, nausea, and vomiting.

❑❑ **What is the physiological reason for Disequilibrium Syndrome?**

During dialysis, excess solutes are cleared from the blood at a faster pace than they can diffuse from the body's cells into the circulatory system.

❑❑ **An M.D. orders "pin care" on a client with skeletal traction. What would this entail?**

Cleaning the areas of skin where the pins enter the bone with one-half strength hydrogen peroxide and one-half strength normal saline.

❑❑ **A client with a history of congestive heart failure presents with coarse rales, pink frothy sputum, restlessness, and dyspnea. What would you suspect is the cause?**

Pulmonary edema.

❑❑ **What would be the best position for this client in bed?**

High fowler's position.

❑❑ **During the first hours after a myocardial infarction, why is it important to monitor the patient's ECG?**

Arrhythmias are the leading cause of death following an infarct.

❑❑ **Four days post-op, a patient has an elevated temperature. This in an indication of what?**

Infection.

❑❑ **A client is taking isoniazid (INH) for active TB. You ask if he has had any right upper quadrant pain. Why?**

INH can cause liver dysfunction in some cases.

❑❑ **A patient is started on propylthiouracil (PTU). What is this medication most commonly used for?**

Hyperthyroidism.

❑❑ **The dietitian instructs a patient with chronic obstructive pulmonary disease (COPD) to eat smaller, more frequent meals rather than 3 large ones. Why?**

Digestion of larger meals takes energy that is needed for breathing. COPD clients eat better and tolerate meals if they eat smaller portions.

❑❑ **When assisting an M.D. with a chest tube removal, how should you instruct the patient to breathe?**

Exhale deeply when the M.D. removes the tube.

❑❑ **The M.D. orders the patient with a closed head injury to be placed on a cooling blanket and given antipyretics. What is the rationale behind this?**

Hypothermia decreases brain metabolism and reduces the chances of brain hypoxia.

❑❑ **What is the danger of taking INH and drinking alcohol on a frequent basis?**

Isoniazid related hepatitis.

❑❑ **Following general surgery, a patient states she wishes to lie still to avoid pain and the need for**

pain medication. How should you respond?

Encourage the patient to take the pain medication as ordered and explain the importance of turning, coughing, and deep breathing every 2 hours.

❑❑ **What type of drugs is administered to reduce secretions and minimize spasms of the larynx when a patient is going to surgery?**

Antiemetics.

❑❑ **Your patient is experiencing severe chest pain 2-3 days after surgery. What may have developed?**

Pulmonary embolus.

❑❑ **A client with right lower lobe pneumonia is admitted. Which nursing action takes priority, elevating the head of the bed, or assessing breath sounds?**

Elevating the head of the bed. The patient's comfort and ease in breathing take priority.

❑❑ **What is the basic principle of bladder training for the quadriplegic?**

Setting up a schedule where the patient empties his bladder at the same time every day.

❑❑ **A patient in the ICU with acute pulmonary edema is given IV lasix. How can you best monitor the patient's response?**

Monitor hourly urine output and vital signs.

❑❑ **Following surgery for a total laryngectomy and radical neck dissection, what should be a nursing priority?**

Maintaining a patent airway.

❑❑ **Why should you count a patient's apical pulse before administering digitalis?**

A symptom of digitalis toxicity is a slow pulse.

❑❑ **During chemotherapy, what measures can help prevent stomatitis?**

Good, frequent, oral hygiene using a soft brush and avoiding any foods that could cause injury to the mouth.

❑❑ **What type of diet does a client need to follow with chronic renal failure?**

A low protein, low potassium diet.

❑❑ **Besides diet, what else should be monitored in a patient with chronic renal failure in regards to intake?**

Fluids should be restricted to a prescribed amount usually determined by the M.D.

❑❑ **What are nursing interventions for the elderly person's GI system?**

Good mouth care, healthy diet and bowel habits, regular exercise, and adequate fluid intake.

❑❑ **What are some of the factors that may affect the dietary patterns of the elderly?**

Inadequate cooking facilities.
Physical inability to prepare food.
Reduced income.
Eating alone.
Loss of teeth or poor fitting dentures.
Lack of transportation or delivery service.

❑❑ **A patient in acute renal failure suddenly begins to have an increased urine output of 4-5 liters per day. What phase of acute renal failure is this called?**

The diuresis phase.

❑❑ **Before surgery, a patient expresses his anxiety about the procedure. What should you do?**

It is common for a client to have anxiety preoperatively. Listen to the patient and allow him to express his anxiety. Use basic verbal skills to help reduce apprehension. Further teaching regarding the surgery may also be needed.

❑❑ **Humans develop in a cephalocaudal direction. What does this mean?**

Development progresses from head to toe.

❑❑ **A client is being admitted for bacterial meningitis. What type of room would be the most appropriate?**

A private room to reduce the spread of the infection.

❑❑ **A client with azotemia, hypertension, and fluid overload is given the nursing diagnosis of Potential for Injury. What is the rationale?**

Azotemia can produce confusion and hypertension can produce visual changes which can lead to injury.

❑❑ **What special skin care measures should be taken with the patient undergoing external radiation therapy?**

Cleanse the skin with warm water avoiding the radiation area so as not to remove the markings. Avoid the use of perfumes or powders which can dry and irritate the skin. Avoid exposure to the sun on radiation areas.

❑❑ **At 24 hours post op for repair of a detached retina, the patient begins to have nausea and vomiting. Should you notify the M.D. immediately? If so, why?**

Yes, notify the physician. Nausea and vomiting can be a sign of increased intraocular pressure.

❑❑ **A patient with Addison's disease presents with dehydration. What is the physiologic factor**

behind this disease which would cause this problem?

The mineral-corticoid deficiency causes an increase in sodium, water, potassium, and chloride loss in the urine.

❐❐ **Which electrolyte is lost during diurect therapy?**

Potassium.

❐❐ **Name the 4 techniques of a physical assessment.**

Inspection, palpation, percussion, and auscultation.

❐❐ **When changing the dressing to a venous access device, what important assessment should you make before reapplying the dressing?**

The condition of the access site and any signs or symptoms of infection.

❐❐ **What type of diet has been shown to decrease your chances of colorectal cancer?**

Low fat, high fiber

❐❐ **When delegating responsibilities to other team members, what 2 factors are considered the most important?**

The appropriateness and the fairness of the assignment.

❐❐ **What nursing measures can help to decrease pruritus associated with Hepatitis?**

Tepid baths and lotions.

❐❐ **If a member of the nursing team appears to be under the influence of drugs or alcohol, what action should you take?**

Notify your immediate supervisor and remove the nurse from her assignment.

❐❐ **A client is receiving IV doxorubicin (Adriamycin). Why is it a high priority to frequently assess for signs of IV infiltration?**

Adriamycin is a vesicant that can cause tissue necrosis and damage to nerves and blood vessels.

❐❐ **What should you do if an IV containing a vesicant infiltrates?**

Discontinue the IV and apply ice to the insertion site. This decreases tissue absorption minimizing injury.

❐❐ **Pelvic radiation often causes what changes in bowel movements?**

Frequent, loose bowel movements are common.

❐❐ **What type of diet can help minimize the occurrence of loose stools during radiation therapy?**

A low residue diet.

❑❑ **What change in a patient's urine would cause suspicion of renal or bladder cancer?**
Intermittent hematuria.

❑❑ **Following administration of preoperative medication, you note that a patient has not signed the consent form. What should you do?**

Notify the physician. Always check to make sure consent forms are signed before administering pre-op medications.

❑❑ **What is one of the most reliable methods of client identification?**

Comparison of client ID bands with the chart information. Never rely on the patient as a means of identification. Medications and physical conditions can affect a client's response.

❑❑ **You come upon a family member who is crying after hearing that a patient has a serious illness. How can you best help that family member?**

Allow family members to express their feelings and show empathy without giving false hope. Emotional support from other family members or clergy would also be appropriate if the family desires it.

❑❑ **Following rhinoplasty, you note that the patient is swallowing frequently. What should you be concerned about?**

Postnasal bleeding.

❑❑ **A client is brought to the emergency department with a diagnosis of a right hip fracture. What would be important for you to assess?**

Neurovascular status of the affected extremity.

❑❑ **Trauma victims are often denied narcotics until what condition is ruled out?**

A closed head injury

❑❑ **What is the most common antiarrhythmic agent used for the treatment of PVC's.**

Lidocaine.

❑❑ **The presence of more than 6 PVC's per minute puts the patient at risk for what arrhythmia?**

Ventricular tachycardia leading to ventricular fibrillation.

❑❑ **A client's blood pressure is 150/90 with no previous history of hypertension. The patient asks if he will have to be put on medication. How should you respond?**

A one time elevated blood pressure reading does not indicate hypertension. The patient should have his blood pressure taken several more times before a diagnosis can be made.

❑❑ **Why is mannitol given in the treatment of head injuries?**

It is a powerful diuretic that will help reduce cerebral edema.

❑❑ **What does the term "stroke in evolution" mean?**
A stroke in which neurologic changes continue to occur for 24-48 hours after the initial incident.

❑❑ **What activities should you instruct a patient to avoid following cataract surgery?**

Any activities that would involve foreword flexion of the head and rapid jerky movements such as driving or vacuuming.

❑❑ **A client is brought into the ED with a decreased level of consciousness, a BP of 45/15, shallow respirations, and ventricular tachycardia on the monitor. What should you do first?**

Prepare to defibrillate the patient and call for help in resuscitation.

❑❑ **After a patient is brought back to a normal sinus rhythm following defibrillation, what medication will most likely be ordered?**

IV lidocaine bolus and an infusion begun.

❑❑ **Why should distilled water not be infused?**

It is a hypnotic solution; this would cause the cells to swell and burst.

❑❑ **Following a myelogram using a water-based dye, you elevate the patient's head and instruct him to drink plenty of fluids. What is the rationale for this?**

Keeping the head elevated will pool the dye in the lower end of the spinal column and decrease irritation to the meninges. Forcing fluids will help replace the cerebral spinal fluid.

❑❑ **What simple assessment indicates that a 3 chamber water seal chest tube is functioning?**

There should be fluid fluctuation with each breath in the water seal chamber.

❑❑ **You dipstick the diabetic client's urine and it tests positive for acetone. What does this indicate?**

The development of ketoacidosis resulting from the body's breakdown of fats.

❑❑ **A client with right-sided hemiplegia following a stroke is most likely to have difficulty seeing objects to which side of the body?**

The right side.

❑❑ **Difficulty speaking and understanding speech if often associated with a stroke to which hemisphere of the brain?**

Left.

❑❑ **What types of foods should the patient avoid 24 hours prior to an EEG?**

Any stimulants, such as coffee or tea.

❒❒ A client with COPD needs oxygen. Which of the following would deliver the most accurate concentration of oxygen: nasal prongs, simple face mask, or venturi mask?

A venturi mask.

❒❒ You note that a patient with hypoxemia is diaphoretic and the skin is cool to the touch. Is this an early or late sign of hypoxemia?

A late sign

❒❒ What electrolyte can become depleted when a patient is on lasix therapy?

Potassium

❒❒ A client suddenly loses consciousness and collapses. What should be your first action?

The first step in basic life support is to assess the level of consciousness by shaking the shoulders and shouting, "Are you okay?" or the patient's name.

❒❒ After you determine the patient to be unresponsive, what is your next step?

Call for help and then begin assessing the "ABC's" - airway, breathing, and circulation.

❒❒ The daughter of a client with rheumatoid arthritis is concerned that she may also develop the disease. What should you tell her?

There is some evidence that there can be a genetic link to the disease, so her concern is warranted. She should follow up with a physician if she desires.

❒❒ You are ordered to start an IV on a client with a low platelet count. What special precautions should you take?

Hold pressure on all unsuccessful venipuncture sites for 10 minutes, use a small gauge IV catheter, wrap the area with gauze to preserve skin integrity, and observe for any bleeding around the puncture site.

❒❒ A client is concerned when she palpates several tender round masses in her breasts before her menstrual period. How should you respond?

These masses are most likely fibrocystic breast nodules. Have her perform the exam after her period to determine if the masses remain the same.

❒❒ What can you recommend when assessing the home of an elderly person for safety?

Walking devices.
Grab bars in the bathroom.
Removal of area rugs and sharp edged furniture.
Appropriate lighting.

❒❒ A client complains of abdominal discomfort and has a palpable bladder, but is voiding only

small amounts at request intervals. What would be the best nursing intervention?

Obtain an order for urinary catheterization. The patient most likely has overflow retention of urine.

❑❑ **When giving discharge instructions to a client with Hepatitis B, you instruct the patient to watch for signs of increased fatigue, nausea, vomiting, and bruising. Why?**

These symptoms could indicate that the patient is having a relapse of the disease.

❑❑ **How long must a client wait after having Hepatitis B before he or she may donate blood?**

A patient who has had Hepatitis B is barred for their lifetime from giving blood.

❑❑ **Two days following hip replacement surgery, a patient is getting out of bed and suddenly complains of severe pain to the surgical site. What should you do?**

Assess the surgical site for any change in the wound, and assess the hip and extremity for a possible dislocation.

❑❑ **What changes in urine output would you expect after administering vasopressin?**

Decrease in urine output for up to 24-96 hours.

❑❑ **A trauma victim is brought into the ED following a MVA. A physician diagnoses a C-4 fracture and suddenly the patient's BP drops and his pulse slows. What could be a possible cause for these symptoms?**

Spinal shock related to the spinal cord injury.

❑❑ **Following a pneumonectomy, which position would be best for a patient?**

Supine (or on the operative side) with the head of the bed elevated.

❑❑ **Approximately 4-6 hours after a patient experiences angina, you receive lab test results revealing that the CPK-MB is elevated. The patient is in no pain at present on a telemetry unit. What should you do?**

Notify the M.D. immediately of the lab results and request that the patient be moved to a cardiac care unit. The patient has had a myocardial infarction.

❑❑ **What are some of the common adverse effects of tamoxifen that the patient should be taught?**

Vaginal bleeding, hot flashes, and weight gain.

❑❑ **A patient with a history of asthma who is taking theophylline is admitted for wheezing. The patient's theophylline level comes back at 6 mcg/ml. Is this normal?**

Therapeutic theophylline level is 10-20 mcg/ml.

❑❑ **You instruct a patient with multiple sclerosis (MS) that it is okay to attend aerobic classes, but she should stop before she becomes fatigued. What is the rationale?**

Clients with MS may exercise, but fatigue can exacerbate their symptoms.

❐❐ **What should be the maximum rate of O2 received by a nasal cannula?**

No more than 6 liters a minute.

❐❐ **The nasal cannula delivers what O2 concentration?**

24-40%.

❐❐ **One hour after extubation, the physician orders arterial blood gasses and wants to be called if they are abnormal. The ABG's are as follows: pO2: 90, pCO2: 40, pH: 7.36. Should you notify the physician?**

No. These are normal.

❐❐ **What is the normal pH of the body?**

7.35-7.45.

❐❐ **Following a stapedectomy, you assess the patient by asking if he can smile. What is the rationale?**

You are assessing the function of the facial nerve (VII). This surgery can result in injury to the facial, acoustic (VIII) or vagus (X) nerves.

❐❐ **A client is admitted with pneumonia and the M.D. orders sputum cultures to be obtained before antibiotics are begun. The patient is unable to cough up any sputum. What should you do?**

Obtain an order to have a sputum sample induced with an aerosol treatment. If still unsuccessful, notify the M.D.

❐❐ **A homeless client complains of night sweats, fever, cough, hemoptysis, pleuritic chest pain, and had a positive PPD skin test. What conclusions can you draw from this data?**

That the patient had been exposed to M. tuberculosis. Diagnosis of active TB is confirmed by chest x ray and sputum samples.

❐❐ **After an injection of edrophonium, (Tensilon), you note that a patient's muscular strength improves. What disorder does this client have?**

Myasthenia gravis.

❐❐ **Following a thyroidectomy, the M.D. orders an emergency tray to be kept at the bedside post-op. What tray could this be?**

An emergency tracheostomy tray. Hemorrhage and respiratory obstruction are complications of this surgery.

❐❐ **A patient with a femur fracture becomes restless, confused, irritable, and experiences dyspnea on the second post-op day. What condition should you assess for?**

Fat emboli syndrome.

❑❑ **Following a stapedectomy, you instruct the patient not to walk unassisted. What is the rationale?**

Following a stapedectomy, the patient can experience vertigo and is at risk for falling.

❑❑ **An M.D. orders streptokinase for treatment of an MI. What is the most harmful complication of this medication that you should assess for?**

Bleeding.

❑❑ **Following a femoropopliteal bypass, you frequently assess pulse, skin color, temperature, and pain on the affected side. What is the rationale?**

A high priority should be placed on detecting the patency of the graft. Any symptoms of occlusion should be reported immediately.

❑❑ **A client is brought to the ED with a C-6 neck fracture. In what position should the patient be maintained?**

Supine with the head and neck midline and immobilized.

❑❑ **Following a transsphenoidal hypophysectomy, you note clear drainage in the dressing, which forms a halo. What is the source of this drainage and what does it indicate?**

The patient is losing cerebral spinal fluid and the M.D. should be notified.

❑❑ **You note a cessation of fluctuation in the water seal bottle from a chest tube. What is the most likely cause?**

Chest tube obstruction.

❑❑ **What must you confirm before administering morphine sulfate?**

The patient's respirations must be above 12.

❑❑ **What is the rationale for the above action?**

Morphine sulfate, like other opiates, can depress the respiratory center.

❑❑ **Which of the following foods contains the highest amount of potassium: corn flakes, whole wheat bread, milk, a baked potato, or an orange?**

A baked potato.

❑❑ **You come upon a COPD client who previously was stable and now complains of dyspnea, his color is dusky, and his skin is cool and clammy. What nursing actions should be taken first?**

Further assess the patient's condition, including vital signs, to determine the best course of action.

❑❑ **Your patient has a diagnosis of right-sided heart failure, what should you monitor?**

Lung sounds, fluid intake, edema of the extremities, and daily weight.

❑❑ **Prior to her cataract surgery, the patient asks you if she can be awake during the surgery and not feel any pain? How should you respond?**

The nerves around and behind the eyes are paralyzed with a local anesthetic.

❑❑ **Why is it important not to give a COPD client high concentrations of oxygen?**

It will depress the COPD client's drive to breathe.

❑❑ **Following a rhinoplasty, you place the patient in the semi-fowlers position. What is the rationale?**

It reduces edema to the surgical area.

❑❑ **What is the mode of transmission for the tubercle bacillus?**

Inhalation of tubercle-laden droplets.

❑❑ **A patient complains stating that when he takes his sublingual nitroglycerin, he gets a burning sensation under his tongue. What is your response?**

This is normal. If this sensation does not occur, then the medication is stale.

❑❑ **To prevent against a patient's nitroglycerin tablets from going stale, how often should they be replaced?**

Every 6 months.

❑❑ **Following casting, what would be the first symptom that would alert you to possible compartment syndrome?**

Pain.

❑❑ **You instruct a patient taking pilocarpine hydrochloride for glaucoma to refrain from driving at night. What is the rationale?**

Pilocarpine is a miotic that can induce impaired night vision.

❑❑ **Following rhinoplasty, you instruct the patient not to drink using a straw until the doctor states it is OK. Why?**

The pressure created when using a straw can initiate bleeding.

❑❑ **What test can you perform to determine if the drainage from the nose following brain surgery is cerebrospinal fluid?**

Test the fluid for glucose using a test strip.

❐❐ What is the basic principle of diet and insulin management in a diabetic who is an athlete?

Increase the intake of carbohydrates and insulin before prolonged exercise.

❐❐ You note that there is no bubbling in the suction compartment of the water seal container of a chest tube. What would be your best course of action?

Check the order to see if the chest tube is ordered with suction and how much. If suction is ordered, increase the suction to the amount ordered.

❐❐ A client calls you and states that she has chest pain, feels short of breath, is sweaty, nauseated, and has a history of heart problems. What should you do?

Tell the patient to hang up and call 911. There is no way to tell for sure, but the patient is describing symptoms of a heart attack which could be life threatening.

❐❐ T/F: Cancer is the leading cause of death in the U.S.

True.

❐❐ In what 4 specific areas does cancer tend to occur?

Lungs, colon, breast, and prostate.

❐❐ You have an order for dry dressing to the RLE. What is the RLE?

Right lower extremity.

❐❐ Before giving a patient his insulin, you remove it from the refrigerator one-half hour before administration. What is the rationale?

Administration of cold insulin promotes lipodystrophy.

❐❐ Why is the administration of propanolol hydrochloride (Inderal) used cautiously in clients with COPD?

It can cause airway resistance.

❐❐ Why should you assess for digitalis toxicity when a patient is taking Lanoxin and lasix?

Lasix decreases the serum potassium level which can increase the toxic effects of digitalis.

❐❐ The patient seems depressed and refuses to participate in his physical therapy because he is "too tired". What would be your best course of action?

Allow the patient to express his feelings and then validate them. This will encourage the patient to talk about his feelings further.

❐❐ What cardiac abnormality can occur with theophylline levels above 35 mcg/ml?

Ventricular arrhythmias.

❑❑ **What physical findings are typical for a patient with a hip fracture?**

The leg on the affected side is usually shorter, it is abducted and externally rotated, and pain is present.

❑❑ **What would be some of the clinical manifestations of esophageal varices?**

Abrupt massive hemorrhage and hematemesis.

❑❑ **What is the most common complication of esophageal varices?**

Esophageal rupture with massive hemorrage and death.

❑❑ **Following a bronchoscopy, the patient is positioned on the side and kept NPO. Why?**

The patient has no gag reflex due to the anesthetic spray used on the back of the throat, therefore, they are at risk for aspiration.

❑❑ **What type of lab study is used to determine if the tubercle bacilli is present in sputum?**

Acid-fast staining.

❑❑ **A patient wants to change to another room because he is afraid that being in room 13 will keep him from getting well. What should you do?**

Move the patient. His fear, even though they might be unfounded, could impede his recovery. Not taking his fear seriously could cause him to lose faith in the medical staff.

❑❑ **What is the recommended site for taking a client's temperature when he is having difficulty breathing and has a productive cough?**

The rectum.

❑❑ **Following a pulmonary lobectomy, you note a decrease in blood pressure, the patient is restless, short of breath, and the chest tube drainage has become sanguineous. What should you suspect?**

Possible internal bleeding at the surgical site.

❑❑ **What changes in chest shape would you expect in someone with advanced COPD?**

An increased anterior-posterior diameter.

❑❑ **A client is admitted with pneumonia. Prior to starting antibiotics, what lab tests should you check?**

Check the results of all cultures obtained.

❑❑ **Before you administer any pain medication, for what should you check?**

When any previous pain medication was given and recent vital signs.

❑❑ **A common adverse effect of aminoglycoside therapy is what type of neurological damage?**

Damage to the 8th cranial nerve.

❐❐ **What advice should you give to a patient who is on oral birth control and is also taking INH?**

An alternate method of birth control should be used. INH decreases the effectiveness.

❐❐ **You would expect an increased amount of calcium to be lost from the body in a bedridden client. Why?**

With decreased activity, calcium is lost from the bones and it is excreted. Osteoporosis often results.

❐❐ **Following a lung lobectomy, you assess the incision line and feel a crackling sensation. What is this called?**

Subcutaneous emphysema.

❐❐ **What should you do if you find subcutaneous emphysema?**

Keep track of its progression. If it spreads rapidly or involves the neck area, it should be reported. Otherwise it poses no danger and is normal after this type of surgery.

❐❐ **What is a hallmark lab sign of ARDS (adult respiratory distress syndrome)?**

Refractory hypoxemia. The PaO_2 level continues to fall despite administering higher levels of oxygen.

❐❐ **Following removal of a chest tube, what should be placed over the wound?**

A petrolatum gauze dressing.

❐❐ **What type of breath sounds will you hear when a pneumothorax is present?**

No breath sounds.

❐❐ **Approximately how many milliliters of fluid are in one unit of packed red blood cells?**

250.

❐❐ **What is the purpose of aminophylline in a patient with COPD?**

To relax and dilate the bronchi and relive bronchial constriction and spasm.

❐❐ **A client taking streptomycin begins to complain of vertigo, tinnitus, ataxia, and hearing loss. Are these symptoms related to the administration of this drug?**

Yes. Aminoglycosides can cause 8th cranial nerve damage which these symptoms indicate.

❐❐ **A client who is perspiring a great deal is at risk for which electrolyte imbalance?**

Hyponatremia.

❐❐ **What is the overall goal for the nursing diagnosis of Impaired Gas Exchange?**

To promote optimal respiratory ventilation.

❒❒ **You note a patient's WBC count to be 13,000/mm3. Is this normal?**

A normal WBC count should be 5,000-10,000/mm3.

❒❒ **What level should the collection and suction bottles from a chest tube be kept at in relation to the patient?**

Below the level of the patient's chest.

❒❒ **Above what level of oxygen concentration is there an increased risk for causing oxygen toxicity?**

40%.

❒❒ **What is the primary reason for infusing a unit of blood over 2-3 hours in a stable client?**

To prevent pulmonary edema.

❒❒ **What is the primary risk factor in the development of COPD?**

Cigarette smoking.

❒❒ **Before administration, what common side effect of atropine sulfate should you mention to the patient?**

Dry mouth.

❒❒ **An M.D. prescribes bed rest for a patient with pneumonia. What is the rationale behind this?**

To reduce the body's demand for oxygen and promote rest.

❒❒ **You should put a high priority on what aspect of teaching in regards to a TB client who is being discharged on medication?**

Take the medication exactly as prescribed.

❒❒ **A patient has an intravenous catheter, what should be assessed?**

The color, location, and appearance of the site.

❒❒ **Can you start an IV in the foot of a patient?**

Yes, if ordered by the physician.

❒❒ **Following a lung lobectomy, the patient is given the diagnosis of Impaired Gas Exchange. What factor is most likely to contribute to this problem?**

Incisional pain decreasing the patient's ability to cough, turn, and adequately breathe deep.

❒❒ **Once a client has had active tuberculosis, at what times in their life are they at risk for**

recurence of the disease?

During highly physical and emotional stress.

❑❑ **What technique can you teach a patient in an effort to reduce the pleuritic pain associated with pneumonia?**

Splint the rib cage when coughing.

❑❑ **What is the single most effective way to reduce the spread of microorganisms?**

Hand washing frequently.

❑❑ **What conclusion can be drawn from a PaO_2 level of 50 in a client that exhibits no signs or symptoms of hypoxia?**

The arterial blood gas is not truly arterial.

❑❑ **A patient with a chest tube following a pneumothorax becomes increasingly dyspneic, tachycardic, and tachypneic. What should you check for?**

Any signs that may indicate that the chest tube is blocked.

❑❑ **Following administration of pain medication, what is an important nursing action that should be done in regards to pain management?**

Assess the effectiveness of the medication.

❑❑ **During the rehabilitation period following chest surgery, you instruct the patient to raise the arm on the affected side over the head. What is the rationale for this exercise?**

To prevent a "frozen shoulder" by maintaining range of motion.

❑❑ **Why is pursed-lip breathing taught to clients with emphysema?**

It causes an increase in the alveolar pressure making it easier to empty the alveoli and eliminate carbon dioxide.

❑❑ **In a patient with bacterial pneumonia, how could humidified air aid in improving the gas exchange?**

It could help to liquefy lung secretions, making them easier to cough up and thus help to clear the airways.

❑❑ **What is the cause of pleuritic chest pain in pneumonia?**

Friction between the pleural layers caused by movements in the chest during inspiration and expiration.

❑❑ **Why are clients often prescribed at least 2 drugs for the treatment of tuberculosis?**

It helps in reducing the development of resistant strains of the disease.

❑❑ **When giving an intradermal injection, what position should the bevel of the needle be in?**

Facing up.

❑❑ **Describe the action of Colace (docusate sodium).**

It is a laxative that allows fluid and fatty substances to enter the stool, thereby softening it.

❑❑ **What groups of people are at a high risk of developing tuberculosis today?**

The elderly, homeless, immunosuppressed/ immunocompromised, foreign born from underdeveloped countries, and substance abusers.

❑❑ **What is the purpose of postural drainage?**

It allows the secretions to move from the smaller airways to the larger airways.

❑❑ **Is it best to use postural drainage before or after chest percussion and why?**

After. Chest percussion helps to loosen secretions so they drain easier.

❑❑ **What medication can help prevent the development of peripheral neuropathies in patients on INH therapy?**

Vitamin B-6 (pyridoxine).

❑❑ **What is an early behavioral sign of hypoxia?**

Anxiety.

❑❑ **What measure can help prevent a reoccuence of bacterial pneumonia in the elderly?**

An annual influenza and pnuemovax vaccine.

❑❑ **Why would it be important for the COPD client to maintain a high fluid intake if no cardiovascular or renal disease is present?**

To help loosen lung secretions so they may be coughed up.

❑❑ **What is the best advice you can give to help patients prevent lung cancer?**

Encourage clients to stop smoking.

❑❑ **What percentage of lung cancer in men and women has been linked to smoking?**

Over 80%.

❑❑ **You should teach a patient with COPD to exhale as they are lifting heavy objects. Why?**

The patient with COPD needs to conserve energy. Exhalation takes less energy than inhalation, so more energy can then be used to perform the task.

❑❑ You note that a patient has developed scattered crackles bilaterally several days following surgery. The patient is instructed to cough and take deep breaths more frequently. What is the rationale?

The patient may not be clearing his airways effectively, especially if deep breathing and coughing causes pain. Instructing the patient to do this more frequently will help.

❑❑ What nerve has the potential to be damaged when a tracheostomy tube is in place?

The laryngeal nerve.

❑❑ What is the most important nursing goal for a client with a new tracheostomy tube?

Maintain a patent airway.

❑❑ A client's serum CPK-MB is elevated. What should you suspect?

Myocardial infarction.

❑❑ Describe some of the commons signs of cardiogenic shock.

Low blood pressure, oliguria, crackles in the lungs, rapid and weak pulse, and diminished blood flow to the brain.

❑❑ What is the rationale for giving morphine sulfate to a client in acute congestive heart failure?

It helps to alleviate the anxiety caused by pulmonary edema and hypoxia.

❑❑ Following heart surgery, it is contraindicated to place the patient's legs in a flexed position, or to place anything behind their knees while lying supine. Explain the rationale.

It may cause pooling of blood in the lower extremities, thus decreasing circulation.

❑❑ A patient comes back from surgery with a NG tube in place. The IV fluids will likely continue until what happens with the NG tube?

No more drainage is returning from the tube.

❑❑ What is your nursing responsibility for evaluating the NG tube?

Check placement every 4 hours. Observe for proper drainage. Measure and record the amount of drainage.

❑❑ T/F: A thrombus is a moving blood clot.

False.

❑❑ T/F: A hemorrhage may be internal or external.

True.

❑❑ **What type of weather tends to aggravate angina pectoris?**

Cold weather.

❑❑ **What environmental factors contribute the most to coronary artery disease?**

Diet.

❑❑ **How soon should you expect to see the effect of lasix, following IV administration?**

5 minutes with a peak effect in 30 minutes.

❑❑ **Following heart surgery, your client experiences persistent bleeding from the incision site. What drug will the physician most likely order to help stop this bleeding?**

Protamine sulfate to reverse heparin.

❑❑ **What important side effect of Inderal (propranolol hydrochloride) should you assess for?**

Slowed pulse rate and associated dyshythmias.

❑❑ **You instruct your client to never stop Inderal abruptly. Why?**

Rebound hypertension may occur.

❑❑ **You are administering an injection at the ventrogluteal site. What is the best position for the patient to prevent discomfort?**

Lying on the abdomen with the toes pointed inward to promote gluteal relaxation.

❑❑ **What blood test can help determine if your client's intake of protein is adequate?**

Serum albumin.

❑❑ **The percent of red blood cells is measured by what lab test?**

Hematocrit.

❑❑ **What is the correct compression rate for 2 man CPR in an adult?**

80-100 per minute.

❑❑ **When administering blood to a client, what type of reaction should you always assess for?**

Anaphylaxis, hemolytic transfusion reactions, bacteremia, and fluid overload.

❑❑ **What are the toxic effects of vitamin B-12?**

B-12 does not have any toxic effects. Any reaction seen is usually related to the substances it is mixed with.

❑❑ **What is believed to be the last of the senses to function in an unconscious client?**

Hearing.

❑❑ **A patient enters the ED with a possible MI and he is in acute pain. The physician orders lab work, an ECG, chest x-ray, and Morphine sulfate for pain. What should be your priority?**

Administering the morphine to relieve the pain.

❑❑ **What are some of the toxic effects of lidocaine?**

Confusion, dizziness, tremors, blurred vision, tinnitus, numbness and tingling of the extremities, hypotension, convulsions, and coma.

❑❑ **What is the mechanism of action of lidocaine upon heart tissue?**

It decreases automaticity of the His-purkinje fibers and raises the stimulation threshold in the ventricles.

❑❑ **A patient on hydrochlorothiazide works at a job where much bending, crouching, and standing is required. Knowing this, what should you assess this patient for?**

Postural hypotension. It is a possible side effect of hydrochlorothiazide.

❑❑ **How can you determine if the chest pain a patient experiences is due to angina or a myocardial infarction?**

Anginal pain is usually relieved by resting, lying down, and/or by administering nitroglycerin.

❑❑ **What is the cause of pain in a myocardial infarction?**

Oxygen deprived ischemic cardiac muscle.

❑❑ **You instruct a patient on prolonged bed rest to frequently move his legs. What is the reason for this?**

To prevent thrombophlebitis and clot formation.

❑❑ **How many pounds are in 1 kg?**

2.2 pounds per kg.

❑❑ **What is the basic principle of behavior modification?**

Behavior is learned and continues when it is rewarded.

❑❑ **Why is it best to instruct a patient to take oral lasix in the morning rather than before going to bed?**

If taken at night, the patient will have to get up several times to void.

❑❑ **What technique is most effective in preventing infection when performing an aseptic procedure?**

Thorough hand washing prior to the procedure.

❐❐ During mitral valve stenosis, blood is unable to fully empty into the left ventricle thereby causing back up of blood from the left atrium into what vessel?

The pulmonary vein.

❐❐ Which lab test is used to determining the dosage of warfarin (Coumadin)?

PT prothrombin time.

❐❐ What vitamin can decrease the anticoagulant effect of warfarin (Coumadin)?

Vitamin K.

❐❐ A patient on a heparin drip is to be switched to oral warfarin (Coumadin). The physician orders warfarin (Coumadin) therapy to begin 36 hours before the heparin is discontinued. Why?

It takes 36-72 hours for Coumadin to take effect.

❐❐ List some risk factors that predispose a patient to atherosclerosis.

Smoking, high cholesterol levels, hypertension, family history, diabetes, obesity, males, and physical inactivity.

❐❐ When applying nitroglycerin paste, what should you avoid?

Getting the paste on your own skin.

❐❐ T/F: Your patient with a diagnosis of Type I diabetes mellitus will require insulin.

True.

❐❐ What information does an ECG provide?

It reflects the electrical impulses transmitted through the heart and can be an indicator of the functional status of the heart muscle and contractile responses of the ventricles.

❐❐ A patient receiving chemotherapy asks why he has to receive 3 different drugs at once. What is generally the reason for this?

The drugs have a synergistic effect on each other when given at the same time.

❐❐ How should you position a patient before beginning CPR?

On a firm surface, on his back.

❐❐ What is the primary physiological alteration that occurs with shock?

Inadequate tissue perfusion.

❑❑ **What activity level would you expect from a patient with iron deficiency anemia?**

Low activity level due to the decrease in the oxygen-carrying capacity of the hemoglobin.

❑❑ **What clinical sign usually causes a patient with Hodgkin's disease to seek treatment?**

Cervical lymph node enlargement.

❑❑ **What is the most common reason a nurse would avoid taking care of terminally ill patients?**

They have not explored their own feelings related to death and dying.

❑❑ **The relative of a terminally ill patient becomes angry and expresses his frustration over the family member's illness. How should you respond?**

Allow the relative to express his feelings, as this is part of the grieving process.

❑❑ **If the chest wall fails to rise during rescue breathing, what could be the cause?**

Airway obstruction, caused by a foreign body, or the head not in the proper position.

❑❑ **When is it acceptable to discontinue CPR?**

When the rescuer is exhausted, the physician orders it to be discontinued, or there is another rescuer available to continue CPR.

❑❑ **What is the primary reason for an IV ordered at a "keep open" rate?**

To provide an emergency route for drugs.

❑❑ **What is the main goal of therapy for a patient in congestive heart failure?**

Increase cardiac output.

❑❑ **What childhood illness can often lead to valvular disease as an adult?**

Rheumatic fever or bacterial endocarditis.

❑❑ **A chest tube accidentally becomes disconnected when the patient turns over in bed. What should you do first?**
Reconnect the tube or place in a bottle of normal saline.

❑❑ **A patient who operates machinery is placed on methyldopa (Aldomet) for hypertension. What should you teach the patient about this drug?**

It can often cause drowsiness and interfere with concentration during the first few days of therapy, so caution should be taken at work.

❑❑ **What is the purpose of a cardiac catheterization?**

To assess the extent of coronary artery blockage.

❒❒ **How can percutaneous transluminal coronary angioplasty cause a fluid volume deficit?**

The contrast medium used can act as an osmotic diuretic and diuresis can result.

❒❒ **Upon what criteria should you base a patient's physical ability for increased activity following a myocardial infarction?**

How easily he tires or shows signs of dyspnea, tachycardia, or fatigue.

❒❒ **What is the best method of evaluating whether oxygen therapy is effective for a patient?**

Arterial blood gases.

❒❒ **What electrolyte imbalance can cause digoxin toxicity?**

Hypokalemia.

❒❒ **Why is it important to instruct a patient with mitral valve stenosis about proper dental care?**

To reduce the risk of bacterial endocarditis resulting from invasive dental procedures or dental infections.

❒❒ **Why is hypertension so difficult to detect in the general population?**

It is basically asymptomatic unless the blood pressure rises to dangerous levels.

❒❒ **How should a patient be instructed to store his nitroglycerin?**

In a tight, light-resistant container.

❒❒ **If a patient receiving chemotherapy develops nausea and vomiting, what would be a priority nursing diagnosis?**
Alteration in nutrition to less than the normal daily body requirements.

❒❒ **Following CPR, a patient regains consciousness. What emotional state is he likely to be in?**

Confusion, anxiety, and disorientation. You should offer emotional support and orient the patient as best as possible.

❒❒ **How can you determine if the fluid replacement therapy administered to a dehydrated patient was effective?**

The urine output is the most sensitive indicator of hydration. It should amount to 30 cc per hour minimum for adequate hydration.

❒❒ **In the absence of renal or cardiac problems, what should be the normal urine output in a patient who is adequately hydrated?**

30-35 ml/hour or greater.

❒❒ **What are the most common sites for bone marrow biopsy in the adult?**

The iliac crest and the sternum.

❑❑ **During rescue breathing in CPR, how is the patient able to exhale?**

Passive relaxation of the chest will force air out naturally.

❑❑ **The physician orders nitroglycerin, and so you obtain an IV infusion pump for administration. What is the rationale for this?**

The infusion pump will ensure that the medication is titrated accurately.

❑❑ **What vital sign should be monitored closely during administration of nitroglycerin?**

Blood pressure.

❑❑ **What is the primary cause of decubitus ulcers?**

Unrelieved pressure over an area leading to poor tissue perfusion.

❑❑ **Why should you take extra precautions regarding skin care when a patient's skin is edematous?**

The potential for skin breakdown is higher because of poor circulation to the tissues.

❑❑ **What should be done if premature ventricular contractions (PVC's) at a rate of 8-10 per minute are noticed on a patient's monitor?**

Notify the physician. PVC's greater that 5-6 per minute are considered dangerous.

❑❑ **What wave is usually indistinguishable on the ECG when atrial fibrillation is present?**

The "P" wave.

❑❑ **How could a patient's pulse be described if atrial fibrillation is present?**

Irregular with a variable rate.

❑❑ **In a patient taking Quinidine, Lasix, and Digoxin, what is a potential side effect of combining these medications?**

Digoxin toxicity. Lasix can cause hypokalemia leading to toxicity, and Quinidine can cause elevated serum Digoxin levels.

❑❑ **What would be an important nursing goal following the insertion of a permanent pacemaker?**

Monitoring the electrical impulse conduction of the heart for stability.

❑❑ **What is the reason that more men than women under 50 years of age suffer from coronary artery disease?**

Estrogen serves as a protection for women from coronary artery disease until menopause.

❑❑ **T/F: Surfactant is secreted from the alveoli located in the upper respiratory system.**

False.

❑❑ **How many lobes do the right and left lungs have?**

There are a total of 5 lobes. The right has 3 lobes and the left has 2 lobes.

❑❑ **Does the pleural cavity contain positive or negative pressure?**

Negative pressure.

❑❑ **Why will a patient with pernicious anemia suffer from B-12 deficiency, even if their diet contains adequate amounts of the vitamin?**

The patient is unable to absorb enough of the vitamin due to an insufficient amount of intrinsic factor in the stomach.

❑❑ **What is the Shilling test?**

It helps to diagnose pernicious anemia by determining the body's ability to absorb B-12 by administering by a radioactive form of the vitamin.

❑❑ **What purpose does protective isolation serve?**

To reduce the transmission of environmental organisms to the patient.

❑❑ **What types of foods are the best sources of B-12?**

Meats and dairy products.

❑❑ **When is it appropriate to administer the Heimlich maneuver on a suspected choking victim?**

Only when the victim cannot make a sound due to airway obstruction.

❑❑ **What would be a priority nursing diagnosis following an MI?**

Impaired Gas Exchange because of the poor oxygenation and dysrhythmias that can occur following an MI.

❑❑ **What would be the purpose of administering digoxin intravenously to a patient with CHF?**

Lanoxin can help strengthen myocardial contractions and thus help increase cardiac output, which will help reduce pulmonary edema.

❑❑ **Following an MI, why is it important to instruct the patient not to reach or strain?**

Reaching or straining could produce the Valsalva maneuver, which could affect cardiac function. Any such activities should be avoided.

❑❑ **What type of diet should a patient be placed on during the acute phase of an MI?**

Small meals, no cardiac stimulants such a caffeine, and avoid foods that can cause constipation.

❑❑ **What type of drug is enalapril maleate (Vasotec), and how does it work?**

It is an angiotensin-converting enzyme (ACE) inhibitor that decreases the level of angiotensin II. This will then decrease peripheral vascular resistance and blood pressure is lowered.

❑❑ **Why is there a potential for blood clot formation in a patient with atrial fibrillation?**

The ineffective contractions of the atria cause blood stasis and thus clot formation.

❑❑ **Prior to a valve replacement, a patient remarks that he hates to take medications and he usually doesn't take what the doctor prescribes for him. Should this statement concern you?**

Following valve replacement, most patients are placed on life long anticoagulant therapy and sometimes antibiotic therapy. Compliance is essential.

❑❑ **According the American Heart Association, what is the definition of hypertension?**

Consistent blood pressure readings of a systolic above 140 and a diastolic above 90.

❑❑ **What is the primary effect of nitroglycerin?**

Peripheral vasodilatation which reduces myocardial oxygen consumption and workload.

❑❑ **What is the most important long-term goal for a patient with hypertension?**

Demonstration of compliance with medication, diet, and exercise regime.

❑❑ **What is a common laboratory finding of the gastric analysis in a patient with pernicious anemia?**

A lack of hydrochloric acid in gastric secretions.

❑❑ **Why would you leave a small air bubble in a syringe before injecting medication?**

To push the medication remaining in the needle into the tissues.

❑❑ **Following chemotherapy administration, a patient begins to vomit. There is no order for an anti-emetic. What should you do?**

Notify the physician.

❑❑ **What is the reason for administering epinephrine to a patient during CPR?**

It stimulates the adrenergic receptors of the heart and can increase impulse conduction, thus stimulating some cardiac activity.

❑❑ **What is the preferred position for a patient who is hypovolemic?**

Flat, with the legs elevated.

❑❑ Why is the Trendelenburg position no longer recommended for hypovolemic shock?

It has been shown to inhibit lung expansion and may increase intercranial pressure.

❑❑ At what age does Hodgkin's Disease affect most individuals?

Young adults between the ages of 20-40.

❑❑ What should be the depth of compressions in an adult when performing CPR?

1.5"-2".

❑❑ What is considered the maximum amount of time that a person can be pulseless, without CPR, and not experience brain damage?

4-6 minutes.

❑❑ What vital sign is used to determine when a patient is able to increase his physical activity following an MI?

Pulse rate.

❑❑ Why should a patient who has just had an MI avoid the Valsalva maneuver?

It can cause a change in heart rate, arrhythmias, increased intrathoracic pressure, and blood clot dislodgment.

❑❑ What type of activities will cause the Valsalva maneuver?

Bearing down against a closed glottis by vomiting, exertion, coughing, or bearing down during a bowel movement.

❑❑ What do crackles (rales) in the lungs indicate?

The alveoli are filled with fluid.

❑❑ A patient taking Lanoxin complains of anorexia, nausea, and vomiting. What should you suspect?

Digitalis toxicity.

❑❑ What type of visual changes occur with digitalis toxicity?

"Yellow-colored" vision and halos.

❑❑ Following open heart surgery, what types of activities should be avoided to prevent damage to the incision line?

No heavy lifting of anything over 10 pounds for at least one month post-discharge.

❑❑ What are the common side effects of nitroglycerin?

Headache, hypotension, and dizziness.

❒❒ **What is coronary percutaneous transluminal coronary angioplasty (PTCA)?**

A balloon tipped catheter is inserted into the coronary artery and compresses the plaque in hopes of dilating the artery.

❒❒ **When chest pain occurs, what is the time interval for administration of nitroglycerin tablets?**

Immediate administration with subsequent doses at 5-minute intervals until the pain has resolved or a total of 3 tablets have been taken.

❒❒ **What should a patient do if his pain is unresolved after taking 3 nitroglycerin tablets?**

Seek medical treatment immediately.

❒❒ **What is a priority goal for a patient with thrombocytopenia following chemotherapy?**

Prevention of potential bleeding.

❒❒ **What age groups are at risk for septic shock due to infection?**

The very young and the elderly.

❒❒ **What common invasive device is a frequent cause of sepsis in the elderly?**

The Foley catheter.

❒❒ **You determine that a patient is breathless and pulseless. After calling for help and positioning him on his back, what should you do next?**

Open the airway and administer 2 breaths.

❒❒ **What are some of the signs of early septic shock?**

Warm flushed skin, confusion, restlessness, tachycardia, and tachypnea.

❒❒ **As septic shock progresses, how does the skin exam change?**

The skin becomes cool and clammy.

❒❒ **Why is "staging" performed in Hodgkin's disease?**

It determines the extent of the disease and is used as a guide in prescribing therapy.

❒❒ **During CPR in adults, what artery should be used to check the pulse?**

Carotid.

❒❒ **What is a common emotional problem that terminally ill patient's face?**

Feelings of isolation

❑❑ **If cardiac compressions are performed inappropriately, what organ is in danger of being damaged?**

The liver.

❑❑ **What symptoms would you expect to find in a patient who has a perforated duodenal ulcer?**

Abdominal rigidity and tenderness.

❑❑ **Following an upper GI endoscopy, what should you monitor besides the patient's vital signs?**

Return of the gag reflex.

❑❑ **Prior to a cholecystography for detection of cholelithiasis, what allergy should you make sure the patient does not have?**

An allergy to iodine or shellfish.

❑❑ **Following a subtotal gastrectomy, what is the purpose of setting the NG tube to low intermittent suction?**

To prevent pressure on the suture lines from accumulated gas or fluid.

❑❑ **Define hemoptysis.**

Blood in the sputum.

❑❑ **What are some of the common symptoms associated with pancreatitis?**

Intense mid-epigastric abdominal pain radiating to the back with nausea and vomiting.

❑❑ **What is the purpose of administering Pro-Banthine in the treatment of pancreatitis?**

It is an antispasmodic often given along with narcotics to help control pain.

❑❑ **How do smoking and drinking alcohol aggravate the symptoms of a hiatal hernia?**

They reduce esophageal sphincter tone, which can result in reflux.

❑❑ **What is the preferred way to determine if a nasogastric tube has been correctly inserted?**

Instill air into the tube while auscultating over the epigastric area.

❑❑ **What stool color indicates that a patient has bleeding in his upper GI tract?**

Black.

❑❑ **What type of diet is considered best for a patient with a peptic ulcer?**

The patient should eat foods that he/she can tolerate (rather than eliminate specific foods from the diet automatically).

❑❑ **Why would a patient with a common bile duct obstruction be monitored for prolonged bleeding?**

Because if bleeding is present, bile is prevented from entering the intestinal tract, thus preventing the absorption of fat soluble vitamins such as vitamin K, which is necessary for prothrombin formation.

❑❑ **In a subtotal gastrectomy (Billroth II), the stomach contents will bypass what anatomical structure?**

The duodenum and go directly to the jejunum.

❑❑ **Following a subtotal gastrectomy, what type of drainage would you expect from the NGT immediately post-op?**

Some bright red bloody drainage, but not in large amounts.

❑❑ **What lab value would be elevated in a patient with pancreatitis?**

Serum amylase and lipase.

❑❑ **What type of diet is recommended for a patient with chronic pancreatitis?**

A low fat, bland diet.

❑❑ **Define functional assessment.**

Functional assessment identifies the person's level of independence and focuses on abilities rather than disabilities.

❑❑ **T/F: Because an elderly person performs activities of daily living (ADLs), it is assumed that instrumental activities of daily living are performed also.**

True.

❑❑ **What nursing measure will help a patient avoid esophageal reflux while sleeping?**

Sleep with the head of the bed elevated.

❑❑ **Following an upper GI series, why do you administer a laxative?**

This test involves barium, which if not eliminated may cause constipation or an obstruction.

❑❑ **What nursing measure can help alleviate a sore nares when a nasogastric tube is in place?**

Applying a water-soluble lubricant around the tube.

❑❑ **When assessing bowel sounds, why should you auscultate the abdomen before palpation?**

Palpating the abdomen first could affect bowel sounds.

❑❑ **How long should you listen in each quadrant to confirm the absence of bowel sounds?**

5 minutes.

❑❑ **T/F: Daily bowel movements are necessary, and less frequent movements are an indication of constipation.**

False.

❑❑ **Why should a patient with a peptic ulcer avoid smoking cigarettes?**

Nicotine increases the release of gastric secretions.

❑❑ **What is the purpose of a T-tube following a cholecystectomy?**

It maintains patency of the common bile duct and allows bile to spill out of the body until the swelling decreases and the bile can again drain into the duodenum. Without it, the bile may drain into the peritoneal cavity.

❑❑ **What type of solution should be used to irrigate a nasogastric tube and why?**

Normal saline. Usage of hypotonic or hypertonic solutions could cause electrolyte imbalances.

❑❑ **Why should you be concerned if a patient with a nasogastric tube complains of nausea, vomiting and abdominal distention?**

These are the symptoms the nasogastric tube is in place to prevent. It could mean the nasogastric tube is not functioning properly.

❑❑ **What is the major cause of acute pancreatitis in the U.S.?**

Alcoholism.

❑❑ **What is the pathophysiology of pancreatitis?**

Stimulation of pancreatic enzymes causes an autodigestive process of the pancreas to occur.

❑❑ **Why would you instruct a patient with a hiatal hernia not to do any heavy lifting after eating?**

Because increases in intrabdominal pressure caused by heavy lifting can aggravate the symptoms of a hiatal hernia.

❑❑ **What is the purpose of administering aluminum hydroxide (Amphojel) to a patient?**

It is an antacid used in the treatment of gastritis or an ulcer.

❑❑ **What is the primary purpose of maintaining an IV in a patient with a nasogastric tube?**

Fluid and electrolyte balance maintenance and fluid replacement.

❑❑ **A bland diet would not include which of the following: salt, sugar, mayonnaise, coffee, eggs,**

Jell-O, or milk?

Coffee.

❑❑ **Which of the following should have the highest priority after admission for cholecystitis: pain control, admission history and physical, or preparing for further tests?**

Pain control. Priority should always be placed on the patient's comfort and safety.

❑❑ **Following a cholecystectomy, what should be eliminated from the diet for the first few weeks?**

Fat.

❑❑ **How is a patient able to produce bile once his/her gallbladder has been removed?**

The gallbladder does not produce bile, it merely acts as a storage for bile. Once removed, bile flows freely from the common bile duct into the intestine.

❑❑ **You are receiving a report and the nurse stated "The patient has a scissors gait." What would you expect to see?**

Crossed-legged walking.

❑❑ **What would cause crossed-legged walking?**

A disorder of the abductor muscles of the thigh or a deformity of the hips.

❑❑ **If a patient has a high abdominal incision, why might you diagnose him as being at high risk for altered respiratory function?**

Because a patient with this incision would be more likely to avoid coughing and deep breathing due to the pain it would cause.

❑❑ **Why is morphine and codeine contraindicated in the treatment of pain due to pancreatitis?**

They may cause spasm of the pancreatic duct and thus increase pain.

❑❑ **What times of the day should pancreatic enzyme therapy be given?**

In conjunction with meals, as they aid in digestion of proteins and fats.

❑❑ **What is a common side effect associated with the use of the antacid Milk of Magnesia?**

Diarrhea.

❑❑ **A patient asks if he will have to have surgery to correct his hiatal hernia. How should you respond?**

Most patients are managed successfully on medication and diet therapy. Surgery is only performed if medical therapy fails to correct the problem.

❑❑ What is the primary indication for the use of prochlorperazine (Compazine)?

It is used as an anti-emetic.

❑❑ Why is it contraindicated for you to reposition a nasogastric tube following gastric surgery?

You could rupture the suture line.

❑❑ What should be checked when gastric distention is noted in a patient with a nasogastric tube?

The suction machine (to ensure it is working properly), the patency of the tube and connections, and the tube's placement.

❑❑ Why does a patient with cholecystitis exhibit nausea, vomiting, and abdominal discomfort after eating a high fat meal?

The digestion of fats is impaired due to the insufficient flow of bile from the gall bladder.

❑❑ When is the best time of the day to administer cimetidine (Tagamet) to a patient?

During meals.

❑❑ What is the function of cimetidine (Tagamet)?

Decrease gastric acid secretion by blocking the H2 receptor in the stomach.

❑❑ What is the correct procedure for recording T-tube drainage?

Record it as output in a separate column from other forms of output.

❑❑ What is steatorrhea?

Diarrhea with fat in the stool.

❑❑ Your patient's blood gas test comes back and shows a high level of CO2. What is the term for this?

Hypercapnia.

❑❑ When the CO2 increases in the tissues and the O2 decreases, your patient may die. What is the term for this condition?

Asphyxia.

❑❑ What symptoms would alert you to a possible leak from the anastamosis site following a partial gastrectomy?

Pain, fever, and abdominal rigidity. Symptoms of peritonitis.

❑❑ What is dumping syndrome?

Following a gastric resection, the patient is at risk for this syndrome in which food moves rapidly from the stomach to the duodenum or jejunum without adequate digestion.

❒❒ **What are some of the symptoms of dumping syndrome?**

Faintness, weakness, dizziness, diarrhea, excessive perspiration, and a bloated feeling.

❒❒ **What diet adjustments can be made to avoid some of the symptoms of dumping syndrome?**

Reduce fluids and carbohydrates. Proteins are allowed because they digest slowly.

❒❒ **What electrolyte imbalance is a complication of pancreatitis?**

Hypocalcemia.

❒❒ **If pancreatic enzyme replacement therapy is inadequate, what change in stool could you expect?**

Steatorrhea.

❒❒ **What symptoms would you expect to find in a patient with a hiatal hernia?**

Heartburn is the most common complaint, with regurgitation and dysphagia also present.

❒❒ **What is the purpose of metoclopramide hydrochloride (Reglan) in the treatment of a hiatal hernia?**

It increases sphincter tone and promotes gastric emptying.

❒❒ **What is the purpose of an incentive spirometer when used post-operatively?**

To prevent atelectasis by promoting deep breathing.

❒❒ **What is the primary reason for withholding food and fluids prior to surgery?**

To prevent the possibility of aspiration of stomach contents during surgery.

❒❒ **When using the ventrogluteal site, what muscle is injected?**

Gluteus minimus.

❒❒ **What is the normal range for a serum potassium level?**

3.5-5.5 mEq/L.

❒❒ **How does castor oil act as a laxative?**

It breaks down in the intestines into ricinoleic acid, which irritates nerve endings causing the evacuation of stool.

❒❒ **What is the primary reason for irrigating a colostomy?**

To stimulate peristalsis so the colon will empty naturally.

❑❑ **What color would the stoma be if it had an inadequate blood supply?**

Dark red to purple. The stoma should be a healthy pink color.

❑❑ **What is the major cause of cerebrovascular accidents in the elderly?**

Hypertension.

❑❑ **What are the most common vision-related pathologic conditions in the elderly?**

Cataracts, glaucoma, and diabetic retinopathy.

❑❑ **T/F: Intelligence decreases with age.**

False. The response time is slower, but the accuracy is greater.

❑❑ **Why is it important for the elderly to exercise?**

To increase cardiac output which will lower blood pressure.

❑❑ **What is the mode of transmission for Hepatitis B?**

Contact with blood or body fluids contaminated with the hepatitis B virus.

❑❑ **What would be the best position for a patient to lie in immediately following a hemorrhoidectomy?**

He should lie prone or on his side to avoid putting pressure on the operative site.

❑❑ **What type of diet will produce stools that will not be as irritating to inflamed hemorrhoids?**

A low roughage, high fiber diet.

❑❑ **What is the cause of a patient's complaint of itching when cirrhosis of the liver is present?**

Increased bilirubin levels.

❑❑ **What type of intestinal obstruction would most likely be present if a patient is vomiting profusely?**

A small-bowel obstruction.

❑❑ **What is the purpose of a Cantor, Harris, or Miller-Abbott tube?**

These are 6-10 foot tubes inserted nasally into the intestines to accomplish decompression when an obstruction is present.

❑❑ **What is the purpose of a Sengstaken-Blakemore tube?**

Used in treating esophageal varices, this tube has a gastric balloon that anchors and applies pressure to the cardiac sphincter and a larger esophageal balloon that that applies pressure to the bleeding sites in the esophagus. Aspiration of stomach contents with a syringe and irrigation is still possible.

❑❑ **What is the difference between an ileostomy and a colostomy?**

An ileostomy is an opening from the ileum (small intestine), and a colostomy is an opening from the colon (large intestine).

❑❑ **When should a patient with an ileostomy empty the pouch?**

When the bag is one-third full or whenever the bag is full enough to cause a break in the seal.

❑❑ **What is the hardest part about having an ileostomy?**

Finding shoes to match the bag.

❑❑ **Why is the use of a skin barrier so important when caring for an ileostomy?**

The drainage from the ileostomy is irritating to the skin due to the high amount of digestive enzymes present.

❑❑ **What is the purpose of administering kanamycin prior to colon surgery?**

To reduce the bacterial count in the colon.

❑❑ **When administering blood, what solution should be administered along with the blood in a tandem set-up?**

Normal saline.

❑❑ **A nasogastric tube is placed following colostomy surgery. When will the physician most likely order it removed?**

When flatus or stool are passed from the colostomy and bowel sounds have returned.

❑❑ **How is Hepatitis A transmitted?**

The oral-fecal route.

❑❑ **What type of precautions should a patient with Hepatitis A be placed on?**

Enteric precautions.

❑❑ **What is the physiological reason for jaundice in Hepatitis?**

Liver inflammation obstructs the normal flow of bile, thus the bilirubin levels rise in the blood causing jaundice.

❑❑ **What is the prophylactic treatment for Hepatitis A?**

Immune serum globulin.

❑❑ **What groups of people are at high risk for Hepatitis B exposure?**

IV drug users, multiple sex partners, health care workers exposed to blood, and homosexuals.

❑❑ **What would the appearance of stools be in a patient with ulcerative colitis?**

Bloody diarrhea stools.

❑❑ **During an acute exacerbation of ulcerative colitis, how is nutrition maintained if a patient is kept NPO?**

Total parenteral nutrition (TPN).

❑❑ **During TPN administration, why would you test a patient's urine regularly for glucose?**

TPN is a hypertonic glucose solution. The urine is tested to evaluate glucose metabolism. Insulin may be required if too much glucose is excreted.

❑❑ **A patient with a potential surgical abdomen complains of abdominal pain upon admission to the ED, but the physician refuses to administer pain medication until his/her abdomen is assessed. What is the reason for this?**

Narcotics may mask symptoms of pain, which is often used as an indication of the severity of the patient's condition.

❑❑ **Why is a Cantor tube not taped in place after insertion?**

It is not taped until it has reached the obstruction. Once in the duodenum it is advanced at a specified rate, allowing peristalsis to carry it through the intestines.

❑❑ **What is the physiological reason for the development of ascites in cirrhosis?**

Portal hypertension and low levels of serum albumin leading to decreased colloidal osmotic pressure and sodium retention, thus fluid leaves the intravascular space and collects in the interstitial space.

❑❑ **Which type of diuretic will facilitate sodium excretion and potassium retention?**

A potassium sparring diuretic such as spironolactone (Aldactone).

❑❑ **What is the danger of the gastric balloon rupturing or deflating in a Sengstaken-Blakemore tube?**

The esophageal balloon can move up, obstructing the airway.

❑❑ **What is the purpose of lactulose (Chronulac) administration in cirrhosis?**

It decreases ammonia formation in the intestine by increasing intestinal motility and causing diarrhea.

❑❑ **A patient with ascites would receive serum albumin for what purpose?**

To increase the colloidal osmotic pressure so fluid will flow from the tissues back into the intravascular space.

❒❒ **What effect would you see if the administration of serum albumin has been successful?**

An increase in urine output as fluid leaves the tissues and returns to the plasma.

❒❒ **What is the purpose of administering oral neomycin and/or neomycin enemas to a patient who has cirrhosis?**

The neomycin helps decrease the amount of bacteria in the intestines. This will produce ammonia as a by-product of digested blood.

❒❒ **What is portal systemic encephalopathy?**

A toxic effect on the central nervous system resulting from the liver's inability to detoxify ammonia.

❒❒ **In what position should you place a patient before administering an enema?**

The left lateral position so the sigmoid colon is below the rectum.

❒❒ **Why should injectable diazepam (Valium) not be mixed with other drugs or solutions prior to injection?**

It is insoluble in water and does not mix with other medications. If mixed it crystallizes.

❒❒ **What are some common symptoms of hyperthyroidism?**

Insomnia, nervousness, tachycardia, muscle tremors, weight loss, and increased appetite.

❒❒ **What complication can occur if the parathyroid glands are accidentally removed during a thyroidectomy?**

Tetany. This is due to the disruption in calcium metabolism (hypocalcemia).

❒❒ **Following a thyroidectomy, what nerve are you testing if you ask the patient to speak?**

The laryngeal nerve. Damage to this nerve is a potential complication following thyroid surgery.

❒❒ **Overproduction of what hormone would result in galactorrhea?**

Prolactin.

❒❒ **Lack of what hormone will cause Addison's disease?**

Adrenocortical hormone.

❒❒ **What types of metabolic imbalances would you expect to find with Addison's disease?**

Hypoglycemia, hyponatremia, hyperkalemia, and dehydration.

❒❒ **What is the mechanism of action for the oral hypoglycemic tolbutamide (Orinase)?**

It stimulates the pancreas to release insulin and increases the number of insulin receptors in the body.

❒❒ **Should an elderly person increase their calcium intake?**

Yes. Calcium intake should be increased to equal 3-4 glasses of skim milk daily.

❒❒ **What dietary products can you recommend to increase calcium intake?**

Cheese, yogurt, milk, and canned salmon with bones.

❒❒ **Why must diabetic patients be concerned about foot care and skin infections?**

The diabetic's ability to heal is compromised along with impaired circulation and decreased sensation to the extremities.

❒❒ **Where would you expect the incision site to be following a transsphenoidal hypophysectomy?**

Between the upper lip and the gums.

❒❒ **What hormone would be present in excess amounts in a 24-hour urine collection from a patient with Cushing's syndrome?**

Cortisol.

❒❒ **What physical symptoms would you expect in a patient with Cushing's disease?**

Skin bruising, muscle wasting, thinning hair on the scalp with increasing amount of hair on the rest of the body, weight gain with a round "moon" face, and fluid retention.

❒❒ **What is the purpose of radioactive iodine therapy in a patient with hyperthyroidism?**

It damages the thyroid tissue so lesser amounts of hormone are secreted.

❒❒ **What types of medication taken prior to a radioactive iodine uptake test could give false positive results?**

Those medications containing iodine taken within the past month.

❒❒ **When do most ethical dilemma typically occur?**

When deciding end-of-life issues.

❒❒ **What effect do foods high in fiber have on blood glucose levels in the diabetic?**

They tend to diminish the rise in blood glucose after meals.

❒❒ **Following a subtotal thyroidectomy, you periodically slip a gloved hand behind the patient's neck. What is the rationale for this action?**

Assessment of post operative bleeding.

❒❒ **How many calories are delivered in one liter of D_5NS?**

170 calories.

❑❑ **How does the body's need for insulin change during times of illness for a patient with insulin dependent diabetes mellitus (IDDM)?**

They increase. A diabetic's glucose level should be monitored closely in times of illness or stress.

❑❑ **Why will a patient who has just had a transsphenoidal hypophysectomy also have an incision on his leg?**

The dura is often closed with a piece of fascia, or muscle, taken from the patient's leg.

❑❑ **What organ is most commonly affected by the vascular changes that occur with long-term diabetes mellitus?**

The kidneys.

❑❑ **What is the best indication that a patient with Addison's disease is receiving the correct amount of glucocorticoids?**

Daily weights as a means of detecting fluid imbalance. Rapid weight gain could indicate fluid retention and hormone replacement therapy would need to be adjusted.

❑❑ **What medication is administered to reverse the effects of diabetes insipidus?**

Vasopressin (Pitressin).

❑❑ **What factors are most important when selecting a needle length for IM injections?**

The amount of adipose tissue present at the injection site and the angle of injection.

❑❑ **What factor determines the needle diameter when preparing an injection?**

The viscosity of the medication.

❑❑ **Why is a patient with Cushing's syndrome at risk for developing kidney stones?**

Calcium loss from the bones increases calcium in the urine leading to calcium deposits in the kidneys.

❑❑ **Diabetes Insipidus is caused by a malfunction of what structure in the brain?**

The pituitary gland.

❑❑ **Define ADL.**

Activity of daily living. These are daily routine functions, such as teeth brushing, hair combing, and face and hand washing.

❑❑ **What is the common term for an acute coryza?**

The common cold.

❏❏ **What is the primary cause of coronary artery disease?**

Cholesterol and other fatty substance within the lining of the artery.

❏❏ **What electrolyte and fluid changes would you expect in a patient with syndrome of inappropriate antidiuretic hormone (SIADH)?**

Hypervolemia and dilutional hyponatremia due to an excess of antidiuretic hormone (ADH).

❏❏ **What eye problem is most often related to long-term diabetes mellitus?**

Diabetic retinopathy.

❏❏ **Why should hypoglycemia be considered dangerous and treated immediately?**

It can lead to brain damage, coma, and even death.

❏❏ **In a patient with Addison's disease, which situations may require an increase in glucocorticoid dosage?**

Illness, severe stress, surgeries, and injuries.

❏❏ **Oral glucocorticoids should always be taken with food for what reason?**

They are very irritating to the stomach and may produce ulcers.

❏❏ **How often should you evaluate a patient's level of comfort when using a patient controlled analgesia system?**

At least every 2 hours.

❏❏ **Following an adrenalectomy for the treatment of Cushing's Syndrome, you are concerned about a patient's incision line, and you monitor it closely. Why?**

Excess cortisol levels over a long period can damage the collagen tissues and impair wound healing. Infection is also a possible complication.

❏❏ **What is the typical treatment for pyelonephritis?**

Antibiotics for 2-4 weeks with a urine culture prior to starting therapy.

❏❏ **What is a common and potentially dangerous complication of peritoneal dialysis?**

Peritonitis.

❏❏ **What is the purpose of giving aluminum hydroxide (Amphojel) to a patient with chronic renal failure?**

It binds phosphates in foods and is administered with or immediately after meals.

❏❏ **What are the 3 different categories of acute renal failure?**

Prerenal, intrinsic, and postrenal.

❒❒ **Why are patients with chronic renal failure often nauseated?**

The presence of retained waste products in the body often causes nausea.

❒❒ **Acute renal failure caused by an obstruction in the urinary tract would be what category of renal failure?**

Postrenal.

❒❒ **Why do patients with chronic renal failure often have dry itchy skin?**

Uremia due to the retention of nitrogenous wastes.

❒❒ **What would be a priority nursing action if disequilibrium syndrome occurs during dialysis?**

Slow the rate of dialysis.

❒❒ **What symptoms would a patient exhibit if disequilibrium syndrome was occurring during dialysis?**

Nausea, vomiting, headache, dizziness, seizures, and confusion.

❒❒ **What should be a priority nursing goal for a patient with renal calculi?**

Relieve the patient's pain.

❒❒ **Where is the best place to secure a Foley catheter to prevent irritation?**

To the inner thigh. The male patient may also have the Foley secured to his abdomen.

❒❒ **What is the purpose of administering the drug allopurinol (Zyloprim) to a patient?**

It reduces uric acid formation responsible for gout and some types of kidney stones.

❒❒ **How long should a patient take antibiotics when being treated for a urinary tract infection?**

As with all infections, this patient should be instructed to take the medication until it is all gone, not just until he/she begins to feel better.

❒❒ **What are some of the common symptoms of cystitis?**

Dysuria, hematuria, burning upon urination, urgency and frequency.

❒❒ **A patient has an order for NPO after midnight the day before surgery. Why is this?**

To prevent aspiration of gastric contents during surgery.

❒❒ **On the morning of surgery, a patient does not want to take her wedding ring off. What could**

you do to ensure sterility in the OR?

Cover the ring with tape.

❒❒ **When starting an IV, at what point in the procedure should you remove the tourniquet?**

After the needle is in the vein.

❒❒ **What serum blood test is the best indicator of renal function?**

Serum creatinine.

❒❒ **What is the most common symptom associated with bladder cancer?**

Painless hematuria.

❒❒ **What is an ileal conduit?**

A portion of the ileum is used as a diversion for urine to flow from the ureters to an opening in the skin on the surface of the abdomen.

❒❒ **Why is it not unusual to find mucus along with urine from an ileal conduit?**

The urine causes some irritation to the intestinal lining and mucus is produced.

❒❒ **Why would you slightly warm the dialysate solution prior to infusing a peritoneal catheter?**

It helps dilate peritoneal vessels, which will help in the removal of serum urea.

❒❒ **What techniques can you use if the return of the dialysate solution is less than the amount infused?**

Since return is accomplished by gravity, having the patient turn from side to side or gentle pressure on the abdomen may help increase dialysate drainage.

❒❒ **While on oral iron therapy, what changes in stool should the patient expect?**

Dark black stools.

❒❒ **When choosing an initial vein for venipuncture in the arm, what location should you try first?**

Choose the most distal location on the arm as possible, such as the hand.

❒❒ **What symptoms would you expect to find if peritonitis was present in a patient on CAPD?**

Cloudy dialysate fluid returns, hyperactive bowel sounds, abdominal pain, and fever.

❒❒ **What is the purpose of phenazopyridine (Pyridium) in the treatment of cystitis?**

It is used as an analgesic that relieves some of the discomfort associated with cystitis.

❑❑ **Why should a patient be instructed to attach a collection bag to the ileal conduit appliance at night?**

It promotes drainage away from the stoma and thus decreases the chance of urine reflux into the ureters.

❑❑ **What is the best way to obtain a urine specimen from a patient with a Foley catheter?**

Clean the drainage tube collection site with alcohol and aspirate urine from the drainage tube using a sterile needle.

❑❑ **Following a cystoscopy, a patient complains of bladder spasms. You note that his urine is pink tinged. What should you do?**

Monitor him, but keep in mind that these are normal symptoms following a cystoscopy.

❑❑ **Immediately following ileal conduit surgery, what symptoms would a patient exhibit if stomal edema became excessive?**

The urine output would drop to below 30 ml/hr due to obstruction of the stoma.

❑❑ **A physician orders sodium polystyrene sulfonate (Kayexalate). What would be the most likely reason for administering this drug?**

Elevated serum potassium level.

❑❑ **What precautions should you take if a patient's potassium level rises to a dangerous level?**

Place the patient on a cardiac monitor and prepare for the possibility of cardiac arrest.

❑❑ **What are some of the sources of Vitamin A?**

Carrots, sweet potatoes, dark leafy green vegetables, and egg yolk.

❑❑ **What is the most common pathologic condition of the neurological system of the elderly?**

Organic brain syndrome.

❑❑ **You are caring for a patient with chronic renal failure. You have been instructed not to take blood pressure in her right arm. What would be the reason for this?**

The patient most likely has an AV fistula or an external cannula in her right arm for dialysis. The blood pressure should never be taken in that arm because of the damage it could cause to the fistula.

❑❑ **During dialysis, regional anticoagulation is used. What does this mean?**

Heparin is infused for anticoagulation into the dialysis machine to decrease the chance of blood clot formation by the dialysis machine.

❑❑ **What medication is given to normalize the clotting time in a patient receiving dialysis?**

Protamine.

❑❑ **What is the medical goal of acute renal failure?**

Restore fluid and electrolyte balance so the body can achieve normal kidney function.

❑❑ **What is the medical goal of chronic renal failure (CRF)?**

Maintain fluid and electrolyte balance artificially through dialysis for the remainder of the patient's life.

❑❑ **What is the most common cause of cystitis?**

An infection introduced from the urethra.

❑❑ **What side effect of phenazopyridine (Pyridium) should a patient be made aware of?**
Bright red-orange urine results and is no cause for alarm.

❑❑ **What is the simplest way to determine the effectiveness of dialysis?**

Weighing the patient before and after treatment.

❑❑ **Is Milk of Magnesia an appropriate over-the-counter medication for patients with chronic renal failure? Why or why not?**

No. It can lead to magnesium toxicity since the kidneys are not able to excrete it.

❑❑ **What is the advantage of CAPD over hemodialysis?**

CAPD allows the patient to be more independent rather than having to spend several days a week at a dialysis treatment center.

❑❑ **Why is it recommended to take vitamin C along with ferrous sulfate?**

It increases the absorption of iron.

❑❑ **What symptoms can you expect if a patient is hyperventilating?**

Dizziness, carpal-pedal spasms, tachypnea, and tingling in the extremities.

❑❑ **Two days following surgery under a general anesthesia, a patient spikes a fever. What would be the most likely source of infection?**

The lungs due to atelectasis.

❑❑ **If cervical cancer is detected early and treated, what is the chance of survival?**

Nearly 100%.

❑❑ **In what quadrant of the breast do most malignant tumors occur?**

Upper-outer quadrant.

❑❑ **You insert a Foley catheter into a patient with an overdistended bladder, but partially clamp**

the tubing to allow the urine to drain at a slow rate. Why?

Rapidly emptying an overdistended bladder may cause shock and hypotension due to the rapid change in pressure in the abdominal viscera.

❑❑ **What is the purpose of administering zidovudine (Retrovir, AZT) to a patient?**

It interferes with the replication of the HIV virus in hopes of slowing the conversion of HIV to AIDS.

❑❑ **What symptoms would a patient exhibit if she is in the early stages of cervical cancer?**

None. This is why routine pap smears and pelvic exams are important.

❑❑ **What is the most effective means of relieving gas pains following abdominal surgery?**
Ambulation.

❑❑ **Why would it be contraindicated to massage a patient's legs if he is at risk for thrombophlebitis?**

It could dislodge a clot that is already present causing further complications such a pulmonary embolism.

❑❑ **What type of container should be kept at the bedside of a patient undergoing internal radiation therapy for cervical cancer?**

A lead lined container and a pair of long forceps for picking up dislodged radioactive materials.

❑❑ **What would you most likely find upon assessment of a patient with epididymitis?**

Scrotal swelling and severe tenderness.

❑❑ **What sensation in the scrotum does a patient complain of when testicular cancer is present?**

A "dragging" sensation.

❑❑ **Following a mastectomy, what position should the patient's arm be placed in on the affected side?**

Elevated on pillows with the distal portions of the arm higher than the more proximal portions.

❑❑ **What is the best position for self-breast examination?**

Supine with a pillow or towel placed under the side being examined to elevate the chest wall.

❑❑ **In relation to a woman's menstrual cycle, what is the best time for self-breast examination?**

During the first week following menstruation.

❑❑ **What is the function of the prostate gland?**

Provide secretions that aid in the nourishment and passage of sperm.

❑❑ **What hormone is often prescribed following a total hysterectomy?**

Estrogen.

❑❑ **A patient asks what skin related reactions she can expect from radiation therapy. How should you respond?**

Redness, dryness, and darkening of the skin are common reactions. Sometimes desquamation and capillary dilation can also occur. Teaching regarding skin care during the time of therapy should be a nursing priority.

❑❑ **A urinalysis report indicates the presence of red blood cells and white blood cells. What is the most likely cause?**

Urinary tract infection.

❑❑ **Does an elderly person's sense of pain increase or decrease?**

Decrease.

❑❑ **Your elderly resident awakes several times during the night. Is this normal?**

Yes. Elderly persons require shorter periods of sleep.

❑❑ **While assisting the M.D. with a vaginal exam, a painless, moist chancre is found by the physician. What is the most likely cause of this type of lesion?**

Syphilis.

❑❑ **In males, what is the most common symptom that causes patients to seek treatment for gonorrhea?**

Painful urination and mucopurulent discharge.

❑❑ **What is the purpose of a Pap smear?**

To identify atypical cervical cells that may be an indication of pathology.

❑❑ **A physician orders a patient with a vaginal radium implant for cervical cancer to be "out of bed as tolerated." Why should you question this order?**

Strict bed rest is the standard of care to prevent dislodgment or movement of the radium implant.

❑❑ **What is the most common treatment of primary syphilis?**

Penicillin.

❑❑ **What symptoms will the female most often experience with gonorrhea?**

Lower abdominal pain, vaginal discharge, fever, and dyspareunia.

❒❒ **How often should a Pap smear be done according to the American Cancer Society?**

Every 3 years after 3 initial negative annual tests in the absence of risk factors.

❒❒ **Following a radical mastectomy, discharge instructions include avoiding cuts, bruises, and injuries to the arm on the affected side. What is the rationale for this?**

Circulation is impaired to that arm and any injury or infection may become more severe.

❒❒ **What are some of the common side effects associated with internal radium implants used in the treatment of cervical cancer?**

Nausea, vomiting, cramping, and foul vaginal discharge.

❒❒ **Why would you advise a patient not to douche in the 24 hours prior to having a Pap smear?**

Douching can wash away cells and secretions needed for good test results.

❒❒ **A patient is concerned that his body will not have enough male hormones after he has had a left orchiectomy. How should you respond?**

The remaining testicle undergoes hyperplasia and produces enough testosterone to maintain normal hormone levels.

❒❒ **What is the most effective method to help control the spread of HIV in the general population?**

Education regarding the mode of transmission and prevention of HIV.

❒❒ **You are caring for a patient who has undergone surgery with spinal anesthesia. What complication might you expect?**

Respiratory failure from paralysis of the vasomotor nerves in the upper spinal column.

❒❒ **What is the purpose of a drainage tube placed in the incision following surgery?**

Removal of accumulated blood and fluids, which could cause pressure on the incision site or increase the chance of infection.

❒❒ **Following a prostatectomy, a patient has continuous bladder irrigation. What guideline should you use as an indicator for the rate of irrigation?**

If the return is bright red, the flow should be increased. This would indicate the presence of blood and a rapid flow is needed to prevent blood clot formation.

❒❒ **What disease is a woman at risk for developing when she has a history of herpes genitalis?**

Cervical cancer.

❒❒ **Why should you be concerned when a HIV positive patient develops a herpes simplex infection?**

Herpes simplex is one of the AIDS defining illnesses. Its presence could indicate that the patient has converted to AIDS.

❐❐ **How should you assess for a distended bladder?**

Palpate the lower abdomen above the symphsis pubis. A distended bladder will produce an uncomfortable rounded swelling in the lower abdomen above the symphysis pubis.

❐❐ **What is the position most commonly used for vaginal exams?**

Lithotomy.

❐❐ **What disorder is often found in the medical history of males with testicular cancer?**

An un-descended testes was probably evident during childhood.

❐❐ **What is the purpose of performing passive range of motion exercises in an unconscious patient?**

To maintain joint mobility.

❐❐ **What part of the brain is responsible for pain perception?**

The cerebral cortex.

❐❐ **Why would activated charcoal be administered following gastric lavage to an overdose patient?**

To absorb any remaining particles of the medication taken.

❐❐ **Why must a patient with pernicious anemia receive B-12 injections, rather than taking it orally?**

The patient is missing intrinsic factor, which is necessary for B-12 to be absorbed from the GI tract.

❐❐ **Why is patient controlled analgesia more effective than intermittent narcotic administration?**

The patient can control when he gets the medication, which reduces the anxiety and leads to a greater pain tolerance and less medication use.

❐❐ **What is believed to be the cause of pain in migraine headaches?**

Dilation of the cranial arteries.

❐❐ **What factors are likely to cause exacerbation of multiple sclerosis (MS)?**

Any stress, fatigue, or exposure to temperature extremes.

❐❐ **What purpose would the drug baclofen (Lioresal) serve when administered to a patient with multiple sclerosis?**

It is a muscle relaxant used to help relieve muscle spasms common with MS.

❐❐ **What is the classic gait exhibited by a patient with Parkinson's disease?**

A shuffling, propulsive gait.

❒❒ **What are the first 4 things you should do if a patient is having a grand mal seizure?**

Ease the patient to the floor, protect the head, protect him/her from injury, and maintain a patent airway.

❒❒ **Why should a patient who is having a seizure not be restrained?**

Strong muscle contractions could cause the patient to injure himself.

❒❒ **What behavior would you expect from a patient following a seizure?**

The patient is usually disoriented and tired (post-ictal), sleeping for a long period of time.

❒❒ **How do you calculate pulse pressure?**

Diastolic pressure minus systolic pressure.

❒❒ **A widening pulse pressure is an indication of what disorder?**

Increased intercranial pressure.

❒❒ **What respiratory pattern is indicative of increased intercranial pressure?**

Slow, irregular respirations.

❒❒ **If a decubitus ulcer is at risk of occurring, what color will the skin turn when pressure is applied to the area?**

White with delayed capillary refill to the area.

❒❒ **What symptoms are common complaints of patients with cataracts?**

Blurred or hazy vision.

❒❒ **What equipment should be available when you perform oral care on an unconscious patient?**

Suction to prevent aspiration.

❒❒ **What is the most important part of catheter care in regards to preventing infection?**

Cleaning the area around the urethral meatus frequently.

❒❒ **What is the purpose of massaging areas of the skin over bony prominence in the unconscious patient?**

To improve circulation to the area and prevent decubitus ulcers.

❒❒ **According to the gate control theory of pain, where is the location of the regulatory center that controls pain impulses?**

The spinal cord.

❒❒ **What is the correct hand placement for locating the ventrogluteal site for injection?**

The palm should be on the greater trochanter, with the index finger on the anterior superior iliac spine.

❒❒ **What is the purpose of placing ankle high tennis shoes on a patient whom is unable to move his legs?**

To prevent plantar flexion (footdrop) from occurring.

❒❒ **To prevent increased intercranial pressure in a patient with a head injury, what position should the head of the bed be in?**

Avoid neck flexion with the head of the bed elevated 30-45 degrees.

❒❒ **In a trauma victim, what initial assessment should receive the highest priority?**

Establishing an open airway.

❒❒ **What is the recommended technique for testing a patient's gag reflex?**

Touch the back of the patient's throat with a tongue depressor or swab.

❒❒ **What side effects will likely manifest if a patient who is on phenytoin (Dilantin) suddenly stops taking the drug?**

Status epilepticus.

❒❒ **What are some nursing interventions in an elderly person with fragile skin?**

Maintain the integrity of the skin.
Avoid hot water, harsh or deodorant soaps, and rubbing alcohol.
Use creams and lotions as needed.
Use cornstarch instead of powder.
Maintain proper nutrition.

❒❒ **A collection of fluid into the abdominal cavity is termed what?**

Ascites.

❒❒ **What routine post-op instruction is contraindicated in a patient who is at risk for increased intracranial pressure?**

Coughing involved in respiratory care to prevent atelectasis.

❒❒ **What is diabetes insipidus?**

A lack of ADH (anti-diuretic hormone), which causes the patient to be extremely thirsty, produce large amounts of dilute urine, and experience electrolyte disturbances.

❑❑ **What type of seizure would be described as a sudden stiffening of the muscles followed by rhythmic, violent muscle contractions.**

Tonic-clonic, or grand mal seizure.

❑❑ **What is the term for a sensory premonition prior to a seizure?**

An aura.

❑❑ **What is a common oral side effect of long-term phenytoin therapy?**

Overgrowth (hyperplasia) of gingival tissues.

❑❑ **Following a cerebral vascular accident, when should a patient begin rehabilitation?**

Rehabilitation begins as soon as the patient is admitted to the hospital.

❑❑ **When teaching a stroke victim to dress himself, which side should he start on?**

The affected side first.

❑❑ **During stroke rehabilitation, a patient's family members express concern because their father cries a lot and has frequent mood swings. How might you advise the family?**

Tell them that this is a normal side effect of the stroke. Trying to divert the patient's attention rather than ignoring, or trying to find a cause to his sadness will be most effective.

❑❑ **A patient is diagnosed with Parkinson's disease and the family asks how long it will take him to return to normal. How should you respond?**

Parkinson's is a progressive disease of which there is no known cure at present.

❑❑ **When prepping a patient's abdomen, you should do what?**

Remove most of the hairs visible and avoid cutting, nicking, or scratching the skin.

❑❑ **Why should you avoid nicking or cutting the skin?**

To decrease the potential of infection.

❑❑ **What is the best position for an unconscious patient undergoing a gastric lavage?**

Lateral or semi prone.

❑❑ **What is the purpose of administering levodopa to a patient with Parkinson's?**

Decrease muscle rigidity and prevent the development of contractures.

❑❑ **Following universal precautions protocol, how should used needles and syringes be disposed?**

Place the entire needle and syringe in a universal precautions sharps container immediately after it is used.

❑❑ **Is recapping a used needle safe?**

No.

❑❑ **Why is the deltoid muscle usually not the muscle of choice for intramuscular injections?**

It is small and often painful when medication is injected, especially if large amounts of medication are used.

❑❑ **Following a CVA, you note that a patient only eats food on half of his plate. What visual phenomena does he most likely suffer from?**

Homonymous hemianopsia, blindness in half of the visual field. Patients who experience this often ignore what is in the half of the visual field that is absent.

❑❑ **Which of the following foods should be avoided prior to the administration of an EEG: an egg a sandwich, Jell-O, milk, diet- cola, carrots, ice cream, or a poppy seed roll?**

Diet cola, because of the caffeine content.

❑❑ **In an unconscious patient requiring surgery, whom may give consent?**

The closest reliable relative.

❑❑ **A patient was brought to the ED with multiple gunshot wounds. The physician determines that this patient requires emergency surgery, or he will die. However, the patient is unconscious and, therefore, is unable to sign the consent forms. No relatives can be found to give consent either. Can this surgery be performed?**

Yes. If the physician determines that the surgery is necessary to save the patient's life, it can be performed without consent.

❑❑ **Following a head injury, a patient's temperature begins to rise. This would most likely indicate an injury to which area of the brain?**

The hypothalamus.

❑❑ **During a trauma exam, you note that a patient has one pupil that is larger than the other. Pressure on what cranial nerve is involved in producing this symptom?**

The third cranial nerve.

❑❑ **What seizure medication can cause a rash as a toxic side effect?**

Phenytoin (Dilantin).

❑❑ **What is the primary cause of new onset seizures in adults over the age of 20?**

Trauma.

❑❑ **What side of the brain has a stroke most likely affected if a patient has expressive aphasia?**

The left side.

❒❒ **What is the area of the brain that controls expressive speech?**

Broca's area.

❒❒ **Why should glass thermometers never be used in a seizure patient?**

If the patient has a seizure while taking their temperature, they could bite down and cut their mouth on the glass.

❒❒ **An unconscious patient become restless, with regards to the respiratory status. What could this indicate?**

Hypoxia.

❒❒ **Prior to administering a tube feeding, what should you do?**

Confirm tube placement and check for tube feeding residual.

❒❒ **How much tube feeding residual is generally considered acceptable?**
Less than 50% of the previous feeding.

❒❒ **After 4 days of hospitalization, a trauma patient asks for pain medication more frequently, becomes restless, and complains that the pain medication is not helping him as much. What should you do?**

Notify the physician that the patient has developed a tolerance for his pain medication dosage, and request an increase or change in his medication.

❒❒ **What is the medical abbreviation for the left eye?**

OS.

❒❒ **What assessment findings would you expect in a patient who has peripheral vascular disease?**

Extremities cool to the touch, pale or cyanotic, pulses difficult to detect, decreased sensation, and cramping in the extremities after activity.

❒❒ **What is the purpose of a myelogram?**

To determine the location of a herniated disk.

❒❒ **A trauma patient is brought to the emergency department and the physician notices crepitus in the right arm. What does this mean?**

Crepitation is used to describe the feeling of bone fragments rubbing together when a fracture is present.

❒❒ **What joints are most commonly affected in osteoarthritis?**

The weight bearing joints (hips and knees) and the fingers.

❑❑ **How does rheumatoid arthritis differ from osteoarthritis in regards to the joints affected?**

Rheumatoid arthritis affects synovial joints, while osteoarthritis affects weight bearing joints.

❑❑ **Which type of arthritis is associated with an autoimmune inflammatory disorder?**

Rheumatoid arthritis.

❑❑ **If a patient taking a bulk producing laxative does not maintain adequate fluid intake, what is a possible side effect?**

Fecal impaction.

❑❑ **What is a laminectomy?**

A surgical procedure that involves removing a portion of the vertebra (lamina), so the nerve root may be explored and parts of a herniated disc removed.

❑❑ **The physician is to perform a thoracentesis. What will you need to assist the doctor?**

A thoracentesis tray, a bedside table, and a pillow.

❑❑ **What would be some of the nursing interventions during a thoracentesis procedure?**

Reassure the patient, try to provide a calming atmosphere, position the patient, and describe what is to be expected.

❑❑ **Where is the dorsalis pedis pulse palpated?**

Medial aspect of the dorsal surface of the foot.

❑❑ **Immediately following amputation of the lower leg, you notice that there is blood seeping through the patient's bandage. Should the physician be notified?**

Some seepage is normal. Mark the area of drainage and re-check in 10 minutes. If the area has greatly increased, or there are signs of hemorrhage, the physician should be notified.

❑❑ **What is the purpose of traction in regards to a fracture?**

To realign bone fragments.

❑❑ **What does the term "passive immunity" mean?**

The body is given an antibody to the toxin of an organism through passive means such as injection.

❑❑ **What is active immunity?**

The body is given an antigen to an organism that stimulates the body to produce its own antibodies to fight an organism.

❑❑ **What type of infection is produced by clostridium perfringens?**

Gas gangrene.

❑❑ **What is your role in regards to maintaining traction in a patient?**

Make sure the weights hang freely, are properly positioned, and the patient is in the proper position in bed.

❑❑ **A patient has fallen 20 feet. What would be a priority concern before moving this patient?**

Possible spinal cord injury requiring head and neck immobilization.

❑❑ **What is the most common cause of autonomic dysreflexia in a patient with a spinal cord injury?**

Bladder distention.

❑❑ **Which arm muscles are involved in crutch walking?**

The triceps.

❑❑ **What is the purpose of administering trimethobenzamide hydrochloride (Tigan)?**

Tigan is given as an antiemetic agent.

❑❑ **What position is contraindicated for a patient with a herniated disc and why?**

Prone, because hyperextension places the most strain on the spine.

❑❑ **What symptom of aspirin toxicity would the patient most likely complain of first?**

Tinnitus.

❑❑ **What is balanced skeletal traction?**

Pressure and counterpressure weights are positioned so the patient may adjust himself in bed without interfering with the traction pull.

❑❑ **Joint swelling is most often found in which type of arthritis: osteo or rheumatoid?**

Rheumatoid.

❑❑ **What is the easiest method and most effective way to prevent a urinary tract infection in a patient with a spinal cord injury?**

Drink at least 2000 ml/day of fluid.

❑❑ **Why is crossing of the legs contraindicated following hip replacement surgery?**

It causes adduction of the hip, which could result in dislocation.

❑❑ **What times of the day should aspirin be given?**

Since it is a gastric irritant, with meals or immediately following meals is best.

❑❑ **Following a total knee replacement, a patient is placed in a continuous passive motion machine. What is the purpose of this machine?**

To prevent flexion deformities and maintain joint flexibility.

❑❑ **How does obesity affect the development of osteoarthritis?**

Osteoarthritis is a degenerative joint disease caused by the wear and tear on weight bearing joints. Obesity increases this wear and tear, and can worsen osteoarthritis.

❑❑ **Following hip surgery, a patient comes back with a drainage tube attached to suction at the incision site. What is the purpose of this tube?**

To prevent fluid accumulation, which can lead to infection and impede wound healing.

❑❑ **When is it acceptable to remove the weights in balanced skeletal traction?**

Not without a physicians order, unless there is an emergency that warrants removal.

❑❑ **When turning a patient in bed, how can you maximize stability and protect your back?**

Wide based stance, bend at the knees, get as close to the patient as possible, do not use your back to lift, and use the weight of the patient to assist you.

❑❑ **What are some common symptoms of a herniated lumbar disc?**

Back pain relieved by rest, a change in deep tendon reflexes, and activities that increase spinal fluid pressure such as sneezing, coughing, and bending cause increased pain.

❑❑ **Why is crutch walking often an impractical goal for the elderly patient?**

The strength required for crutch walking and the coordination necessary is often impaired in the elderly.

❑❑ **Following a laminectomy, what position must the patient be placed in?**

Any position that maintains the spine in straight alignment avoiding the prone position which could cause hyperextension.

❑❑ **Following limb amputation, the patient complains that he can still feel his missing limb. What is this phenomena called?**

Phantom limb sensations. Real sensations including pain may be present and should be taken seriously and treated accordingly.

❑❑ **What technique should be used when turning a patient who has just had a laminectomy?**

Log rolling.

❑❑ **During rehabilitation, a patient with a spinal cord injury notices muscle spasms in her legs and**

is excited about the return of movement. How should you respond to this finding?

Gently explain to the patient that this is a normal reflex action from the muscles that is uncontrollable by the brain. It is an indication that spinal shock is over, but not an indication that function is returning.

❑❑ **What position should a spinal cord injury patient be in when applying a back brace?**

Lying flat in bed.

❑❑ **Following hip replacement, what precautions should be taken when the patient lies on her side?**

Avoid adduction by placing an abductor splint or pillows between the patient's legs.

❑❑ **How does psyllium hydrophilic mucilloid (Metamucil) help in bowel elimination?**

It creates bulk in the stool by absorbing water and creating a soft, gelatinous substance.

❑❑ **Following a myelogram, why would you encourage a patient to drink plenty of fluids?**

To help replace cerebrospinal fluid, facilitate absorption and excretion by the kidneys of the contrast medium, and to prevent a spinal headache.

❑❑ **What suggestions could you give a patient to protect his skin when he is ordered to wear a back brace?**

A soft cotton T-shirt underneath the brace will keep the brace clean and help to absorb body moisture, while providing protection to the patient's skin. The patient should inspect his skin after removal of the brace for areas of potential skin breakdown.

❑❑ **How long can spinal shock last following a spinal cord injury?**

It can last for several weeks after the initial injury.

❑❑ **T/F: Strict isolation is necessary for the patient with pulmonary TB.**

True.

❑❑ **What are 2 different systems for isolation recommended by the CDC for Isolation Precautions?**

Disease-specific isolation and category-specific isolation.

❑❑ **Approximately one-half hour prior to a dressing change for a burn patient, what nursing action should be performed?**

Administration of the prescribed analgesic. Dressing changes are painful. Patient tolerance and comfort are important when caring for burned tissue.

❑❑ **When performing pin care, should you remove the crusting or scab formation that develops around the pin or should it be left and treated as a wound which is healing?**

Remove the scab formation. It can trap bacteria causing an infection to develop.

❒❒ **Following the amputation of a patient's lower leg, you notice that the patient's surgical site is bleeding. What should you do?**

Notify the physician and apply direct pressure to the site, or apply a tourniquet if the bleeding is profuse.

❒❒ **Why is the spinal cord injured patient at risk for kidney stone formation?**

Lack of weight bearing on the long bones causes bone demineralization and thus more calcium is excreted by the kidneys causing stone formation.

❒❒ **Why does a severe burn patient often receive TPN rather than oral or tube feedings?**

Paralytic ileus is a common result of a severe burn so oral feeding would not be tolerated.

❒❒ **What is the most effective way to evaluate the effectiveness of tracheobronchial suctioning?**

Auscultate the lungs before and after the procedure.

❒❒ **What is eschar?**

Dead burned tissue that is without blood supply, often heavily contaminated with bacteria.

❒❒ **Why are coughing, sneezing, and bending at the waist contraindicated following cataract surgery?**

These actions increase intraocular pressure, which can damage the operative site.

❒❒ **You are present when a person catches on fire. What should you direct the person to do?**

Stop, drop, and roll to extinguish the flames, or cover the person with a large blanket. Do not run.

❒❒ **What is Meniere's disease?**

An inner ear disorder causing tinnitus and vertigo.

❒❒ **How should you first attempt to stop an acute nosebleed?**

Have the patient sit upright, head slightly forward, and pinch the soft tissues of the nose together.

❒❒ **What is the physiological cause of glaucoma?**

An obstruction in the outflow of aqueous humor causes an increase in intraocular pressure. Chronic high pressure can damage the retinal nerve leading to blindness.

❒❒ **What is a retinal detachment?**

The 2 layers of the retina separate at a tear or hole causing vitreous humor to seep into the tear further separating the retinal layers.

❒❒ **What are Curling's ulcers?**

Stress ulcers that can develop as a result of physiological stress from a burn. The chance of these ulcers developing is usually proportional to the extent of the burn.

❑❑ **What is the most common cause of cataracts?**

Aging.

❑❑ **Blood volume makes up what percent of a person's total body weight?**

Approximately 8%.

❑❑ **Where should you instruct a patient who is using crutches to put most of his body weight?**

On his hands. Placing most of the body weight under the arms can cause damage to the axillary nerve.

❑❑ **What is the physiological cause of autonomic dysreflexia?**

The body reacts with a sympathetic response to autonomic nervous system stimulation.

❑❑ **What possible physiological complication of a spinal cord injury should you be aware of in the acute trauma phase?**

Spinal shock.

❑❑ **What causes a patient with a spinal cord injury to become dizzy when positioned in an upright position?**

The lack of vasomotor tone to the lower extremities causes pooling of blood and thus a lower amount of blood returning to the heart, causing hypotension.

❑❑ **What are some common symptoms of autonomic dysreflexia?**

Sudden severe hypertension, a pounding headache, "goosebumps," and profuse sweating.

❑❑ **Traction applied directly to a pin inserted in the bone is an example of what?**

Skeletal traction.

❑❑ **Several days following a femur fracture, the patient develops fat emboli. What are some of the symptoms that he could display?**

Respiratory distress, hypoxia, confusion, or agitation and petechia found over the chest.

❑❑ **What signs would alert you to possible infection at the pin site with skeletal traction?**

Pain, swelling, and redness.

❑❑ **T/F: Infectious diseases are no longer a significant public health problem.**

False.

❏❏ Following cataract surgery, a patient complains of pain in his eye and he appears restless. What potential complication could be occurring?

Intraocular hemorrhage.

❏❏ Following a laryngectomy, what is the priority nursing goal in the immediate post-op period?

Maintain a patent airway.

❏❏ What is the medical treatment for Meniere's Disease?

Many treatments are used including diuretics, antihistamines, anticholinergics, and a low sodium diet.

❏❏ What is the cause of "floaters" commonly seen by patients with a retinal detachment?

Red blood cells that have been released into the vitreous humor.

❏❏ What is the correct site to instill eye drops?

The lower conjunctival sac.

❏❏ What effect does a miotic agent have on the pupil?

It constricts the pupil.

❏❏ What should you do if a patient with Meniere's disease has an acute attack?

Have him lie down in a safe and comfortable position. Do not allow the patient to stand on his or her own to avoid injury.

❏❏ What effect does a mydriatic agent have on the pupil?

It dilates the pupil.

❏❏ Why is it important to administer an antiemetic as soon as the patient complains of nausea following cataract surgery?

Vomiting could increase intraocular pressure.

❏❏ Which 2 common complications should you watch for in a patient who has just undergone nasal surgery?

Airway obstruction and hemorrhage.

❏❏ What is a tonometer?

A device which measures intraocular pressure.

❏❏ What position should a patient be placed in when a retinal tear is present?

The patient's position is determined by the location of the tear. The goal is to have the detached retinal fragment fall back into the correct location.

❑❑ **What complication will result if Meniere's Disease is left untreated?**

Hearing loss.

❑❑ **During the first 48-72 hours following a severe burn, what is the best way to monitor the accuracy of fluid replacement?**

Hourly urine output monitoring is the most reliable indicator of fluid replacement.

❑❑ **Why would you hyper oxygenate a patient prior to suctioning his airway?**

To prevent hypoxia resulting from the suctioning procedure.

❑❑ **Why are a patient's eyes patched when a retinal detachment is present?**

It decreases eye movements that could worsen the detachment.

❑❑ **What is the medical abbreviation for both eyes?**

OU.

❑❑ **What should be included in a patient's discharge plan following cataract surgery?**

The ability to judge distances is impaired so the patient should use caution to avoid injury.

❑❑ **What are the risk factors for developing laryngeal cancer?**

Chronic alcohol use, smoking, or exposure to other noxious fumes.

❑❑ **When bandaging a burn patient's hand, you place gauze between the fingers, which prevents the skin surfaces from touching one another. Why do you do this?**

Because skin surfaces that touch each other can cause irritation and can interfere with healing.

❑❑ **What symptoms does a patient display if he has a retinal detachment?**

Seeing "flashing lights" or "floaters" and a non-painful loss of vision frequently described as "a curtain slowly drawn across the eye."

❑❑ **What is the maximum time that airway suctioning should be performed?**

No longer than 10 seconds.

❑❑ **What type of glaucoma is considered a medical emergency?**

Acute narrow-angle glaucoma.

❑❑ **Following nasal surgery, how should you assess for excessive bleeding?**

Check the back of the throat for bleeding, watch for excessive swallowing, and check the nasal dressing for blood.

❑❑ What is the outcome of an untreated retinal detachment?

Blindness.

❑❑ What should be the temperature of the solution used for ear irrigation?

Body temperature.

❑❑ What is the procedure for the emergency treatment of a burn victim?

Assess the ABCs, apply cool water to the burned area, and remove smoldering clothing.

❑❑ What is an early symptom of laryngeal cancer?

Hoarseness.

❑❑ When suctioning a patient via the trachea or an endotracheal tube, when is suction never applied?

When inserting the catheter into the airway.

❑❑ What are the symptoms of narrow angle glaucoma?

Severe eye pain, rapid vision loss, and colored halos around lights.

❑❑ During burn healing, what nutritional alteration is required?

Increasing the intake of calories and protein.

❑❑ What factors are critical for a successful outcome of a skin graft?

Lack of infection, immobilization of the area, and the development of vascularization to the area.

❑❑ What solution may be instilled into a tracheostomy or endotracheal tube to help liquefy secretions prior to suctioning?

1-2 ml of sterile normal saline.

❑❑ Why should an order for atropine be questioned in a patient with glaucoma?

Atropine causes pupil dilation, which can increase intraocular pressure.

❑❑ What physiological fluid shift would you expect during the acute phases of a burn?

Fluid shifts from the vascular space to the interstitial spaces causing edema and hypotension.

❑❑ Following packing removal from a rhinoplasty, how long should a patient abstain from blowing his nose?

At least 48 hours and then only very gently.

❑❑ **Airway suctioning is considered a clean or sterile procedure?**

Sterile.

❑❑ **What causes the fluid shifts seen in a patient sustaining a burn?**

The damaged cells cause the release of histamine substances, which increase capillary permeability. Thus, fluid leaves the intravascular space and enters the interstitial space.

❑❑ **Why would a patient be fed through a nasogastric tube following a laryngectomy?**

It prevents contamination of the suture line and prevents fluids from leaking though the wound into the trachea.

❑❑ **Why would you place a patient in the semi-fowlers position immediately following nasal surgery?**

It helps decrease swelling, increase comfort, and assist in breathing.

❑❑ **Why would the discharge instructions for a patient treated for scleral buckling include an instruction to avoid reading?**

Reading causes frequent and jerky eye movements, which could inhibit the healing process.

❑❑ **What is the medical abbreviation for the right eye?**

OD.

❑❑ **How can you prevent medication from entering the tear duct when administering eye drops?**

After instilling the eye drop, apply light pressure against the nose at the inner angle of the patient's closed eye.

❑❑ **Why is frequent mouth care important following nasal surgery?**

Mouth breathing dries the oral mucous membranes.

❑❑ **What are the typical criteria for brain death (these may vary from state to state)?**

Unresponsiveness to painful stimuli, absence of spontaneous respiration or muscle movement, and loss of brainstem function (as evidenced by fixed, dilated pupils, and absence of reflexes, and a flat electroencephalogram).

❑❑ **When caring for a patient who is receiving diuretics, what should you monitor?**

Serum electrolytes, vital signs, urine output, and observe for orthostatic hypotension.

❑❑ **A patient with a pressure sore should be on what type of diet?**

High protein, high caloric diet unless contraindicated.

❑❑ **After a 12-hour fast, what should the normal fasting blood glucose level be?**

70-100 mg/dl.

❑❑ **How is the blood pressure reading affected if the blood pressure cuff used is too narrow?**

A falsely elevated blood pressure reading will be obtained.

❑❑ **What result can occur from using a blood pressure cuff that is too wide?**

A falsely decreased blood pressure reading may be obtained.

❑❑ **What are the common complaints of a patient who is suffering from digitalis toxicity?**

Diplopia, blurred vision, light flashes, and yellow-green halos around images.

❑❑ **What is anuria?**

A daily urine output of less than 100 ml.

❑❑ **What test is used to differentiate between sickle cell trait and sickle cell anemia?**

The hemoglobin electrophoresis test.

❑❑ **What are the adverse affects of chemotherapy?**

Bone marrow depression causing anemia, leukopenia, and thrombocytopenia. GI epithelial cell irritation causing mucosal ulcerations, bleeding, vomiting, and destruction of hair follicles and skin causing alopecia and dermatitis.

❑❑ **What type of diet should a patient undergoing chemotherapy consume?**

A high-calorie, high-protein diet.

❑❑ **When should postural drainage be scheduled?**

2-4 hours after meals to reduce the patient's risk of vomiting.

❑❑ **What constitutes a positive Kernig's sign?**

A positive test occurs when an attempt to flex the hip of a recumbent patient produces painful spasms of the hamstring muscles and resistance to further leg extension at the knees.

❑❑ **In what part of the spine do herniated intervertebral discs most commonly occur?**

Lumbar and lumbosacral region.

❑❑ **What is a laminectomy?**

A surgical removal of the herniated portion of an intervertebral disc.

❑❑ **For a patient in cardiac arrest, what is the first priority?**

Establish an airway.

❑❑ **What is the most common symptom of Alzheimer's disease?**

Memory loss.

❑❑ **What is the drug of choice for reducing premature ventricular contractions?**

Lidocaine hydrochloride.

❑❑ **What constitutes a positive tuberculin test?**

10 mm or more of induration at the injection site.

❑❑ **What is the most common finding in a patient with bladder carcinoma?**

Gross painless hematuria.

❑❑ **What does a positive Trousseau's sign indicate?**

Hypocalcemia.

❑❑ **What is required prior to an invasive procedure?**

Informed consent.

❑❑ **What does the drug probenecid (Benemid) do?**

It is given along with Penicillin and delays Penicillin excretion, keeping the antibiotic in the body longer.

❑❑ **What type of ulcer is characterized by pain 2 hours after eating, and is relieved by eating more food, drinking milk, or taking an antacid?**

Duodenal ulcer.

❑❑ **What is the purpose of the Z-track intramuscular injection technique?**

To seal medication deep into the muscle, thereby minimizing skin irritation and staining.

❑❑ **T/F: Evisceration occurs when an incision suddenly opens up and the intestines are released to the outside of the body.**

True.

❑❑ **What type of ulcer is characterized by pain during or shortly after eating a meal?**

Gastric ulcer.

❑❑ **In a patient who cannot void, the first nursing action should be?**

Assess the bladder by palpation.

❒❒ **What are the characteristics of vitamin C deficiency?**

Brittle bones, pin point peripheral hemorrhages, and friable gums with loosened teeth.

❒❒ **What are the 5 stages of the nursing process?**

Assessment.
Nursing diagnosis.
Planning.
Implementation.
Evaluation.

❒❒ **What is the most common fracture in the elderly?**

Hip fracture.

❒❒ **What is the appropriate needle size for an insulin injection?**

25 gauge and 5/8 inch (1.5 cm) long.

❒❒ **What does paroxysmal nocturnal dyspnea indicate?**

Congestive heart failure.

❒❒ **What does the acronym SOAP represent?**

It represents a format used to write nursing progress notes. The S stands for Subjective data; O for Objective data; A for Assessment; and P for Plan.

❒❒ **In the SOAP format, who provides the subjective data?**

The patient.

❒❒ **What are the signs and symptoms of a pneumothorax?**

Tachypnea, restlessness, hypotension dyspnea, and possible hypoxia.

❒❒ **What is the first sign of toxic shock syndrome?**

Rapid onset of a high fever.

❒❒ **What are the signs and symptoms of a perforated peptic ulcer?**

Sudden severe upper abdominal pain, vomiting and a tender rigid abdomen.

❒❒ **What is wasting syndrome?**

The rapid weight loss experienced in a patient with AIDS.

❑❑ **Where is a medulloblastoma characteristically found?**

Cerebellum.

❑❑ **What are the dietary needs of a patient undergoing dialysis?**

Vitamin supplements and foods that are high in calories but low in protein, sodium. and potassium.

❑❑ **In a patient with finger clubbing, what pulmonary condition must be suspected?**

COPD.

❑❑ **What is the most reliable and accurate way to administer oxygen to a patient with COPD?**

Venturi mask.

❑❑ **What is a cataract?**

Opacity of the lens.

❑❑ **Before removing a foreign body from a patient's eye, what should you first check?**

The patient's visual acuity.

❑❑ **What is a chancre?**

A painless ulcerative lesion that develops during the primary stage of syphilis.

❑❑ **You are to perform sensory testing on an 85-year-old person. How should you perform this?**

Use a cotton ball for light touch and a safety pin for deep touch. Touch the skin at different places bilaterally from head to toe while the person's eyes are covered. Ask them to distinguish between light, dull, and sharp.

❑❑ **What is the single best method of limiting the spread of micro-organisms?**

Hand-washing.

❑❑ **What is the most reliable indicator of positive response to therapy during the administration of total parenteral nutrition (TPN)?**

Weight gain.

❑❑ **What is ascites?**

The accumulation of fluid in the abdominal cavity commonly caused by cirrhosis.

❑❑ **What is von Willebrand's disease?**

An autosomal dominant bleeding disorder that results from platelet dysfunction and Factor VIII deficiency.

❒❒ **Describe petechia.**

Tiny, round, purplish-red spots that appear on the skin and mucous membranes as a result of intradermal or submucosal hemorrhage.

❒❒ **What is purpura?**

Any purple skin discoloration caused by blood extravasation.

❒❒ **Why is early ambulation after surgery encouraged?**

To increase peristalsis and stimulate venous circulation.

❒❒ **Should the doctor be informed of the presence of bowel sounds in the post-op patient?**

Yes. This is a positive sign and the patient may have the NG tube removed.

❒❒ **A butterfly rash across the bridge of the nose is a characteristic sign of what connective tissue disorder?**

Systemic lupus erythematosus (SLE).

❒❒ **How long does it take for a cast to dry?**

24-48 hours.

❒❒ **When should a tuberculum skin test be read?**

48-72 hours after administration.

❒❒ **What is the most common transfusion reaction?**

A febrile, nonhemolytic reaction.

❒❒ **Describe a 4-point gait with crutches.**

Patient first moves the right crutch followed by the left foot and then the left crutch by the right foot.

❒❒ **Describe a 2-point gait with crutches.**

The patient moves the right leg and the left crutch simultaneously and then moves the left leg and the right crutch.

❒❒ **When should you avoid taking a rectal temperature in an adult patient?**

Cardiac disease, anal lesions, bleeding hemorrhoids, or recent rectal surgery.

❒❒ **If cyanosis occurs circumorally, sublingually, or in the nail beds, the oxygen saturation is below what level?**

80%.

❐❐ **What is Cullen's sign?**

A bluish discoloration around the umbilicus of a postoperative patient.

❐❐ **What does Cullen's sign indicate?**

Intra-abdominal or peritoneal bleeding.

❐❐ **Before ambulating a postoperative patient, what should you have the patient do?**

Dangle his/her legs over the side of the bed and perform deep breathing exercises.

❐❐ **What are the signs and symptoms of hypovolemia?**

Rapid weak pulse, low blood pressure, cool clammy skin, shallow respirations, oliguria or anuria, and lethargy.

❐❐ **In a postoperative patient, what organism is most likely to cause septicemia?**

E. coli.

❐❐ **What are the signs and symptoms of septicemia?**

Fever, chills, rash, abdominal distension, prostration, pain, headache, nausea, and diarrhea.

❐❐ **What are the 3 names given to all pharmaceutical drugs?**

The generic name, which is used in official publications.
The trade or brand name, which is selected by the pharmaceutical company.
The chemical name that describes the chemical composition of the drug.

❐❐ **What is the most common cancer among men?**

Lung cancer.

❐❐ **What are the characteristics of a tonic-clonic (grand mal) seizure?**

Loss of consciousness with alternating periods of muscle contraction and relaxation.

❐❐ **Who is the ideal donor for a kidney transplant?**

A biological sibling.

❐❐ **What is the most common cancer in females?**

Breast cancer.

❐❐ **Describe the 4 stages of cervical cancer.**

Stage 0: Carcinoma in situ.
Stage 1: Cancer confined to the cervix.

Stage 2: Cancer extension beyond the cervix but not to the pelvic wall.
Stage 3: Cancer extension to the pelvic wall.
Stage 4: Cancer extension beyond the pelvis or within the bladder or rectum.

❑❑ **What are the signs and symptoms of a small bowel obstruction?**

Decreased bowel sounds, abdominal distention, decreased flatus, and projectile vomiting.

❑❑ **When using one hand to ventilate an adult patient with an Ambu bag, how many cc's of air are delivered?**

400 cc.

❑❑ **When using 2 hands to ventilate with an Ambu bag, how much air can be delivered?**

1,000 cc of air.

❑❑ **What are the early indications of gangrene?**

Edema, pain, redness, tissue darkening, and coldness in the affected body part.

❑❑ **What are the findings in a patient with polycythemia vera?**

Pruritus, painful fingers and toes, hyperuricemia, plethora (reddish, purple skin and mucosa), weakness, and easy fatigability.

❑❑ **What are the characteristics of thyroid storm?**

Hyperpyrexia with a temperature up to 106 degrees F, diarrhea, dehydration, tachycardia, arrhythmia, extreme irritability, and delirium.

❑❑ **What is tardive dyskinesia?**

Involuntary, repetitive movements of the tongue, lips, extremities, and trunk.

❑❑ **What are the findings in Grave's disease (hyperthyroidism)?**

Weight loss, nervousness, dyspnea, palpitations, heat intolerance, increased thirst, exophthalmos, and a goiter.

❑❑ **What type of isolation should be used in a patient with measles?**

Respiratory.

❑❑ **A high level of hepatitis B serum marker (HBsAg) 3 months after the onset of acute hepatitis B infection suggestions what?**

The development of chronic hepatitis or a carrier state.

❑❑ **What are the signs and symptoms of aortic stenosis?**

Low blood pressure, angina pectoris, arrhythmias, exertional dyspnea, fatigue, and a loud systolic murmur over the aortic area.

❒❒ **What is the most common administration route for epinephrine?**

Subcutaneous.

❒❒ **What is the most serious complication in a patient who has had an acute stroke?**

Increasing ICP.

❒❒ **What are the signs and symptoms of acute pancreatitis?**

Low grade fever, tachycardia, hypotension, discolored flank (Grey Turner's sign), vomiting, and epigastric pain.

❒❒ **What is "Locked-in" syndrome?**

A complete paralysis caused by brainstem damage. Only the eyes can be moved voluntarily.

❒❒ **After a fracture, what are the stages of bone healing?**

Hematoma formation, cellular proliferation, callous formation, ossification. and remodeling.

❒❒ **After myelography, how long should a patient remain recumbent?**

24 hours.

❒❒ **What is nystagmus?**
An involuntary and rapid horizontal, vertical, or rotatory eye movement.

❒❒ **What is hypothermia?**

A life-threatening disorder in which the body's core temperature drops below 95 degrees F (35 degrees C).

❒❒ **What is the triad of symptoms seen in Reiter's syndrome?**

Arthritis, conjunctivitis, and urethritis.

❒❒ **How often should heel protectors be removed to inspect the foot for signs of skin breakdown?**

Every eight hours.

❒❒ **What are the signs and symptoms of chlamydial infection?**

Urinary frequency, thin white vaginal or urethral discharge, and cervical inflammation.

❒❒ **What is the most prevalent sexually transmitted disease in the U.S.?**

Chlamydia.

❑❑ **What are the signs and symptoms of secondary syphilis?**

Enlarged lymph nodes, alopecia, erosions of the oral mucosa and a rash on the palms and soles.

❑❑ **Define sterilization.**

A process by which living microorganism are destroyed.

❑❑ **How many types of anesthesia are there?**

Two: general and local.

❑❑ **Your patient has dressing changes ordered every shift and prn. What should you observe during the dressing change?**

Color, odor, drainage, and depth.

❑❑ **What complications can occur in a patient taking an MAO inhibitor while consuming a high tyramine diet?**

The patient may experience a hypertensive crises marked by dangerously elevated blood pressure, headache, chills, nausea, and restlessness.

❑❑ **What is the most common postoperative problem?**

Bleeding.

❑❑ **Before administering a medication, what should you do?**

Identify the patient by checking the identification band and asking the patient to state his or her full name.

❑❑ **How should a site for injection be cleaned?**

A sterile alcohol swab should be used and wiped in a circular motion from the center of the site outward.

❑❑ **What should you do if blood is aspirated into the syringe before an IM injection?**

Withdraw the needle, prepare another syringe, and repeat the procedure.

❑❑ **What should you do if bleeding occurs after an injection?**

Apply pressure until the bleeding stops. If bruising occurs, monitor the site for an enlarged hematoma.

❑❑ **What causes varicose veins?**

Valvular insufficiency.

❑❑ **What type of isolation is best for a patient on chemotherapy?**

Reverse isolation, because the WBC count may be depressed.

❑❑ **What type of care instructions should you give to a patient who has had congestive heart failure?**

Take digitalis and other drugs as prescribed, restrict sodium intake, restrict fluids as prescribed, get adequate rest, gradually increase walking and other activities, avoid temperature extremes, report signs of congestive heart failure recurrence, and keep all regular physician appointments.

❑❑ **What are the signs and symptoms of pyloric stenosis?**

Palpable, olive-sized mass in the right upper quadrant; strong, peristaltic movements from the left to right during kneels; and projectile vomiting.

❑❑ **What solution should be used to irrigate a gastric tube?**

Normal saline.

❑❑ **What may hypotension indicate in a patient with an MI?**

Cardiogenic shock.

❑❑ **How does nitroglycerine help relieve the pain associated with angina and an MI?**

It causes coronary artery vasodilatation leading to an increase in blood flow to cardiac muscle.

❑❑ **If a client has ascites from chronic liver disease, what position should help with respiration?**

The Semi-Fowler's position.

❑❑ **What should you do if a continuous total peripheral nutrition (TPN) infusion is abruptly interrupted?**

Administer 5% dextrose in water, at the same rate, because abrupt cessation can result in hypoglycemia.

❑❑ **What blood type is considered the universal donor?**

Type O negative.

❑❑ **What blood type is considered the universal recipient?**

Type AB positive.

❑❑ **How many ECT treatments should a patient receive if they are to be effective?**

6-12 treatments, at a rate of 2 or 3 per week.

❑❑ **What is the drug of choice for treating status epilepticus?**

Phenytoin (Dilantin).

❑❑ **What is the most sensitive test for liver dysfunction?**

Prothrombin time.

❒❒ **What is suggested by a return of brown dialysate during peritoneal dialysis?**

Bowel perforation.

❒❒ **What is the most fatal complication of severe acute pancreatitis?**

Hypovolemia.

❒❒ **What are some of the unalterable risk factors for coronary artery disease?**

Heredity, age, race, and sex.

❒❒ **Describe arterial bleeding.**

Bright red, flows rapidly, and spurts with each heartbeat.

❒❒ **When should penicillin be taken?**

1-2 hours before or 2-3 hours after meals, because food may interfere with the drug's absorption.

❒❒ **What is the normal life span of a RBC?**

110 to 120 days.

❒❒ **What is the most common bacteria involved in urinary tract infections?**

Escherichia coli.

❒❒ **What urine pH level is considered normal?**

4.5 to 8.

❒❒ **What factors can cause a urine pH greater than 8.0?**

Urinary tract infection, high alkaline diet, or systemic alkalosis.

❒❒ **What factors can cause a urine pH less than 4.5?**

A high protein diet, fever, or metabolic acidosis.

❒❒ **What is pulsus alternans?**

A regular pulse rhythm with an alternation of weak and strong beats. It occurs in ventricular enlargement, because the stroke volume varies with each heart beat.

❒❒ **Define cardiac output.**

The amount of blood ejected from the heart per minute. It is expressed as liters per minute.

❒❒ **What is the most common cause of septic shock?**

Gram negative bacteria such as E. coli, Klebsiella pneumonia, and pseudomonas.

❑❑ **How should you position a patient when performing a percutaneous renal biopsy?**

Prone. He should also be on a firm surface, with a sandbag under the abdomen to stabilize the kidney.

❑❑ **What are the characteristics of nephrotic syndrome?**

Proteinuria, hypoalbuminemia, edema, and ascites.

❑❑ **What are the signs and symptoms of toxic shock syndrome?**

Temperature greater than 102 degrees F, rash, systolic blood pressure less than 90 mm Hg, and desquamation of the palms and soles of the feet.

❑❑ **What is a bruit?**

A vascular sound that resembles a heart murmur. It results from turbulent flow through a diseased or partially obstructed artery.

❑❑ **What are the signs and symptoms of toxicity from thyroid replacement therapy?**

Sleep disturbance, dysuria, weight loss, irritability, diaphoresis, and a rapid pulse rate.

❑❑ **What is the most common allergic reaction to penicillin?**

Rash.

❑❑ **T/F: Deep and rapid respirations are an early sign of aspirin toxicity.**

True.

❑❑ **What gauge needle should be used for subcutaneous injections?**

25 gauge needle.

❑❑ **How often should you perform passive range of motion exercises on an unconscious patient?**

Every 2-4 hours.

❑❑ **What does the term "oriented times 3" indicate?**

The patient is alert and oriented to person, place, and time.

❑❑ **What fluids would you monitor when calculating output?**

Urine, vomit, drainage from tubes, blood loss, stool, and perspiration.

❑❑ **How should a patient be positioned after having had a thyroidectomy?**

The patient should remain in a semi-Fowler's position with the head firmly supported by pillows, avoiding neck flexion.

❒❒ **What medication can be given via enema to lower an elevated potassium level?**

Sodium polystyrene sulfonate (Kayexalate).

❒❒ **Where on the body does jaundice first manifest?**

The sclera.

❒❒ **Why should a patient in the acute stage of infectious mononucleosis limit his activities?**

To minimize the possibility of rupturing an enlarged spleen.

❒❒ **How long should you count an irregular pulse?**

60 seconds.

❒❒ **Forwhat is the bell of the stethoscope used?**

To hear low-pitched sounds such as heart murmurs.

❒❒ **What are 2 severe complications of femur fractures?**

Blood loss and fat emboli.

❒❒ **What is dry gangrene?**

Tissue that is uninfected and mummified with a tendency to self-amputate.

❒❒ **What is wet gangrene?**

Tissue that is moist, infected, swollen, and painful. A rapid spread of infection is noted.

❒❒ **What is the purpose of the diaphragm of the stethoscope?**

It is used to hear high-pitched sounds such as breath sounds.

❒❒ **How much of the arm should a blood pressure cuff cover?**

One-third of the patient's upper arm.

❒❒ **How far should the blood pressure cuff be from the antecubital fossa?**

One inch.

❒❒ **What is ptosis?**

Eyelid drooping.

❒❒ **What is the first sign of a pressure ulcer?**

Reddened skin that blanches when pressure is applied.

❒❒ **What is the approximate breathing rate at rest for an adult?**

14 bpm.

❒❒ **A 30-year-old female has been admitted for restrictive disease. What should you monitor?**

Respiration rate.

❒❒ **What are the signs and symptoms of chronic sickle cell anemia?**

Cardiomegaly, systolic and diastolic murmurs, chronic fatigue, hepatomegaly, and tachycardia.

❒❒ **What are the signs and symptoms of early childhood sickle cell anemia?**

Jaundice, bone pain, ischemic leg ulcers, pallor, joint swelling, chest pain, and an increased susceptibility to infection.

❒❒ **What is the definition of drug tolerance?**

The need for increasing amounts of a medication to achieve an effect that was formerly achieved with a smaller dosage.

❒❒ **What is Bell's palsy?**

Unilateral facial weakness or paralysis that is caused by disturbance of the seventh cranial nerve.

❒❒ **T/F: Ethylene chloride is a local anesthetic.**

True.

❒❒ **What are the characteristics of angina pectoris?**

Substernal pain that lasts 2-3 minutes, and may radiate to the neck, shoulders, or jaw. It is usually described as vise-like or constricting pain. It may be associated with diaphoresis, nausea, and a feeling of impending doom.

❒❒ **What is indicated by anginal pain that persists for more than 20 minutes and is not relieved by nitroglycerine?**

A developing myocardial infarction.

❒❒ **What are the signs and symptoms of acute kidney transplant rejection?**

Progressive enlargement and tenderness at the transplant site, increased blood pressure, decreased urine output, fever, and an elevated serum creatinine level.

❒❒ **A patient status post right radical mastectomy may have their blood pressure taken in which arm?**

The left arm.

❒❒ Where should you secure the loose end of a restraint after first attaching it to a bed-ridden patient?

The bed frame or springs.

❒❒ What are the signs and symptoms of theophylline toxicity?

Vomiting, restlessness, tachycardia (greater than 200 beats per minute), sweating, and anxiety.

❒❒ What is considered a normal central venous pressure?

2-3 mm Hg (or 3-15 cm of water).

❒❒ How do you prevent a DVT after surgery?

Subcutaneously administer heparin every 8-12 hours.

❒❒ What condition or complication might you suspect if the daily drainage from a patient's nasogastric tube exceeds 3 fluid liters?

Possible intestinal obstruction.

❒❒ What type of diet should be prescribed for a patient with celiac disease?

A gluten-free diet.

❒❒ T/F: Open-ended questions are best when seeking information from a patient.

True.

❒❒ What is atelectasis?

An incomplete expansion of lung segments or lobules.

❒❒ After a patient has gone into cardiopulmonary arrest, how long does it take for brain damage to occur?

4-6 minutes.

❒❒ Why is milk contraindicated for patients who have ulcers?

Because its high calcium content stimulates secretions of gastric acid.

❒❒ Which protection items should be removed first when leaving an isolation room?

Gloves and gown should be removed before the mask, because the mask carries fewer pathogens.

❒❒ How often should TPN and the setup tubing be changed?

Every 24 hours.

❑❑ **How often should a peripheral IV site be changed?**

Every third day.

❑❑ **What is the reason for providing skin care at skeletal pin insertion sites?**

To prevent osteomyelitis.

❑❑ **How can you tell if a dialysis shunt is functioning properly?**

A thrill can be palpated or a bruit can be auscultated.

❑❑ **What are some of the early physical signs of AIDS?**

Fever, pallor, anorexia, fatigue, night sweats, and large lymph nodes.

❑❑ **If a patient has Alzheimer's disease, what should nursing care focus on?**

The implementation of safety measures.

❑❑ **What is the normal BUN value?**

10-20 mg/dl.

❑❑ **What are the signs of Parkinson's disease?**

Muscle rigidity, a pill-rolling tremor, akinesia, and a mask-like face.

❑❑ **What are the signs and symptoms of a fat embolism?**

Fever, tachycardia, tachypnea, anxiety, and chest pain.

❑❑ **What medication can cause gingival hyperplasia?**

Phenytoin sodium (Dilantin).

❑❑ **Would the cerebral spinal fluid (CSF) protein be high or low in a patient with meningitis?**

High.

❑❑ **What are the adverse effects of epinephrine?**

Palpation, headaches, tachycardia, dyspnea, hypertension, and anxiety.

❑❑ **What are the 3 membranes that enclose the brain and spinal cord?**

The dura mater, pia mater, and arachnoid membrane.

❑❑ **What are the leading causes of blindness in the U.S.?**

Diabetes mellitus and glaucoma.

❒❒ **What is the initial treatment of wound dehiscence?**

Cover the wound with moist sterile dressing and notify the physician.

❒❒ **What are the characteristics of bone pain?**

Deep, intense pain that usually worsens at night and is unrelated to movement.

❒❒ **What are the adverse effects of long-term steroid use?**

Weight gain, headache, fatigue, increased urine retention, and acne.

❒❒ **What are the major hemodynamic changes associated with cardiogenic shock?**

Decreased left ventricular function and decreased cardiac output.

❒❒ **How soon after surgery should a patient void?**

Within 8 hours.

❒❒ **What are the symptoms of a hiatal hernia?**

A feeling of fullness in the upper abdomen or chest, heartburn, and pains that are similar to that of angina pectoralis.

❒❒ **What are the risk factors for cholecystitis?**

A family history of cholecystitis is one factor. Other factors are categorized as the 4 F's: female, fat, 40, fertile (i.e. female, overweight, greater than 40 years of age, and women who have had multiple childbirths in the past).

❒❒ **An acetaminophen overdose can severely damage which organ?**

The liver.

❒❒ **What is the first symptom of pancreatitis?**

A constant epigastric pain that radiates to the back.

❒❒ **What does somnambulism mean?**

Sleep walking.

❒❒ **What is obstipation?**

Extreme intractable constipation caused by an intestinal obstruction.

❒❒ **How often should a rectal tube's balloon be deflated?**

For 20-30 minutes every eight hours.

❑❑ **What is a sarcoma?**

A malignant tumor located in the connective tissue.

❑❑ **What is a reducible hernia?**

A protruding mass that can be placed back into the abdomen.

❑❑ **What is the first step in managing a drug overdose or drug toxicity?**

Establish and maintain an open airway.

❑❑ **How do you remove wax or a foreign body from the ear?**

Gently flush with warm saline solution.

❑❑ **Name 2 symptoms of corneal transplant rejection.**

Eye irritation and decreasing visual fields.

❑❑ **What should be done with the urine of a patient with suspected renal or urethral calculi?**

Strain for calculi.

❑❑ **What are the early signs and symptoms of tuberculosis?**

Low-grade fever, weight loss, night sweats, fatigue, cough, and anorexia.

❑❑ **What are the signs and symptoms of acute rheumatic fever?**
Chorea, fever, carditis, migratory polyarthritides, erythema marginatum, and subcutaneous nodules.

❑❑ **What is the treatment for alcohol withdrawal?**

IV glucose, thiamine, folic acid, and an anti-anxiety medication, such as chlordiazepoxide (Librium).

❑❑ **What is the most common symptom of hepatitis A?**

Anorexia.

❑❑ **How is hepatitis A spread?**

Fecal oral route.

❑❑ **What is phimosis?**

A tightening of the prepuce of the penis, which prevents foreskin retraction over the glands.

❑❑ **The physician has ordered RICE for your patient with a sprained ankle. What does this abbreviation mean?**

Rest, ice, compression, and elevation.

❑❑ **What are the complications associated with aminoglycoside use?**

Nephrotoxicity and ototoxicity.

❑❑ **When testing the 6 cardinal fields of gaze, which cranial nerves are being assessed?**

3, 4, and 6.

❑❑ **What is a hordeolum?**

Infection of one or more of the sebaceous glands of the eyelid.

❑❑ **What is a chalazion?**

An eyelid mass resulting from chronic inflammation of the meibomian glands.

❑❑ **What are some of the causes of a respiratory alkalosis?**

Pulmonary embolism, asthma, severe hypoxia, high fever, and hyperventilation syndrome.

❑❑ **What are the causes of a metabolic acidosis?**

Diabetic ketoacidosis, lactic acidosis, diarrhea, renal failure, toxic drug ingestion, and high doses of acetazolamide.

❑❑ **What does a positive Murphy's sign indicate?**

Cholecystitis.

❑❑ **What are the symptoms of appendicitis?**

Right lower quadrant pain, abdominal rigidity, rebound tenderness, anorexia, and nausea.

❑❑ **A patient with suspected appendicitis states his pain has suddenly dissipated. You call the M.D. immediately. Why?**

You suspect rupture of the appendix.

❑❑ **After abdominal surgery, what should you assess closely in the early post op period?**

The incision site for drainage, bleeding, or swelling. Vital signs should also be monitored to detect any signs of internal bleeding.

❑❑ **What is the major complication of a perforated appendix?**

Peritonitis.

❑❑ **A patient with suspected appendicitis complains of pain, but narcotics may be contraindicated at this time. Why?**

Until the diagnosis is made, pain meds should be avoided because they may mask the symptoms and give false results when examining the patient.

❑❑ **What are some of the complications of gentamycin toxicity?**

Nephrotoxicity and ototoxicity.

❑❑ **A patient with an NG tube complains of nausea. What should you do first?**

Make sure the NG tube is working properly and placement is correct. Irrigate it if necessary to test patency.

❑❑ **What is the function of folic acid and B-12?**

Nuclear protein synthesis and RBC maturation.

❑❑ **What does chest physiotherapy include?**

Postural drainage, chest percussion and vibration, coughing, and deep breathing exercises.

❑❑ **Describe the findings associated with Kawasaki's disease.**

High temperature for more than 5 days, conjunctivitis, strawberry tongue, cervical lymphadenopathy, carditis, rash to the palms and soles of the feet, and red, dry, cracking lips.

❑❑ **What is Cushing's syndrome?**

A disorder resulting from an excessive level of adrenocortical hormones. It is manifested by a moon face, peripheral wasting, acne, mood swings, hirsutism, amenorrhea, and decreased libido.

❑❑ **What is the approximate oxygen concentration of a patient receiving 3 liters of O2 per nasal cannula?**

32%.

❑❑ **What does the term "silent myocardial infarction" indicate?**

An MI that produces no symptoms.

❑❑ **What are the adverse reactions to verapamil?**

Headaches, hypotension, atrial-ventricular conduction disturbances, dizziness, and hypotension.

❑❑ **What activities should you encourage a patient to do after chest surgery?**

Sit upright and perform deep breathing and coughing exercises.

❑❑ **What is the primary reason for treating streptococcal pharyngitis with antibiotics?**

To protect the heart valves and prevent rheumatic fever.

❑❑ **What are the common complications of gastric lavage?**

Vomiting and aspiration.

❐❐ **What is pica?**

A craving to eat non-food items, such as dirt, clay, starch, or hair.

❐❐ **What are the factors that affect the action of a drug on the tissues?**

Excretion, distribution, metabolism, and absorption.

❐❐ **What are the adverse reactions to cyclosporin?**

Renal and hepatic toxicity, GI bleeding, hypertension, confusion, and delirium.

❐❐ **What is a living will?**

A witnessed document that states a patient's desire for certain types of care and treatment.

❐❐ **What are the signs and symptoms of a urinary tract infection?**

Urinary urgency, frequency, dysuria, hematuria, abdominal cramps, and urethral itching.

❐❐ **What is quality assurance?**

A method of determining whether nursing actions and practices meet established standards.

❐❐ **What are the 5 rights of medication administration?**

The right route, the right time, the right dose, the right medication, and the right patient.

❐❐ **What type of diet should be ordered for a patient with Crohn's disease?**

A diet that is low in residue, fiber, and fat, but high in calories, protein, and carbohydrates.

❐❐ **What is the most common site for a pulmonary emboli to originate?**

The leg veins.

❐❐ **What patient care measures should be implemented during a sickle cell crisis?**

Bed rest, IV fluids, oxygen, analgesics, and a thorough documentation of fluid intake and output.

❐❐ **When is a fat embolism most likely to occur after a fracture has been sustained?**

Within the first 24 hours.

❐❐ **What does a CPK-MB level greater than 5% of the total CPK indicate?**

An acute myocardial infarction.

❐❐ **What are the findings in cardiogenic shock?**

Tachycardia, cyanosis, weak pulse rate, diaphoresis, pale cool skin, blood pressure below 80 mm Hg, and oliguria of less than 30 ml of urine per hour.

❑❑ **Name some foods that are high in potassium.**

Watermelon, bananas, oranges, soy beans, and lima beans.

❑❑ **What is Cheyne-Stokes respiration?**

Alternating periods of apnea and deep, rapid breathing.

❑❑ **What is the most common cause of airway obstruction in an unconscious patient?**

The tongue.

❑❑ **What is the chest compression rate for adult CPR?**

80-100 times per minute.

❑❑ **Why would you place a patient on a bland diet?**

To prevent gastric irritation.

❑❑ **What is the problem with a clear liquid diet?**

It is void of all nutrients and can, therefore, only be consumed for a short period of time.

❑❑ **What are Battle signs?**

Bluish discolorations behind the ears of patients who have sustained a basilar skull fracture.

❑❑ **T/F: Superficial pain is usually described as prickling.**

True.

❑❑ **What are Schedule V drugs?**

Medications, such as cough syrups containing codeine, which have a low potential for abuse.

❑❑ **How long should one unit of packed RBC's be administered?**

Over a 2-4 hour period.

❑❑ **What are the characteristics of Schedule I drugs?**

These drugs, such as heroine, have a high abuse potential and have no currently accepted medical use in the U.S.

❑❑ **What is the solvent of the body?**

Saline.

❒❒ A patient requests hot chocolate with breakfast. You check her diet order and find a clear liquid diet is ordered. What should you do?

Suggest an alternative such as hot tea.

❒❒ How should you approach a visually impaired person?

From the front.

❒❒ What steps are involved in obtaining a sputum specimen?

The patient should rinse their mouth with clean water, cough deeply from the chest, and expectorate into a sterile container.

❒❒ How should a patient be positioned after having had a liver biopsy?

The patient should lie on the right side to compress the biopsy site, which will decrease the possibility of bleeding.

❒❒ What are the dietary needs of a patient with cirrhosis?
Low-sodium, high protein diet containing at least 3000 calories per day. The patient should also be placed on daily vitamin therapy.

❒❒ What gauge needle is used to administer packed RBC's or whole blood?

16 or 18 gauge.

❒❒ Why must a large needle be used to administer whole blood or packed RBC's?

To avoid RBC hemolysis.

❒❒ What should you do if a patient feels faint during a bath or shower?

Turn off the water, cover and lower the patient, and summon help.

❒❒ What phenomena is characterized by intermittent ischemic attacks in the fingers and toes, which are marked by severe pallor, paresthesia, and pain?

Raynaud's syndrome.

❒❒ What does the abbreviation D.S. indicate?

Double strength.

❒❒ What is the drug colchicine used for?

To relieve inflammation and treat gout.

❒❒ What infectious organism causes tuberculosis?

Mycobacterium tuberculosis

❑❑ **What does the term "myopia" indicate?**

Nearsightedness.

❑❑ **What is the most common symptom of a pulmonary embolis?**

Chest pain.

❑❑ **If a patient has a conductive hearing loss, in which ear will the sound be heard when performing the Weber test?**

The ear that has the conductive loss.

❑❑ **What is trismus?**

Painful spasms of the muscles of mastication.

❑❑ **What does the term "bradycardia" refer to?**

A heart rate of less than 60 beats per minute.

❑❑ **How far above the stoma should the bag be hung during colostomy irrigation?**

18 inches (45 cm).

❑❑ **What is the mortality rate from receiving contaminated blood?**

50%.

❑❑ **What should be done if a blood transfusion is not started within 30 minutes after the blood has been received from the blood bank?**

Return it to the blood bank, because the refrigeration facilities on a typical nursing unit are inadequate for storing blood products.

❑❑ **What are the factors that affect body temperature?**

Time of day, age, physical activity, and phase of menstrual cycle and pregnancy.

❑❑ **What does the term "stress incontinence" mean?**

Involuntary urine leakage that is triggered by a sudden physical strain such as a cough, sneeze, or quick movement.

❑❑ **What does the term "urge incontinence" mean?**

The inability to suppress a sudden urge to urinate.

❑❑ **What does the term "total incontinence" mean?**

Continuous urine leakage resulting from the bladder's inability to retain urine.

❑❑ **What is gastric lavage?**

The flushing of the stomach and removal of ingested substances through a nasogastric or orogastric tube.

❑❑ **What are the common postoperative complications?**

Atelectasis, pneumonia, thrombophlebitis, pulmonary embolism, septicemia, and hypovolemia.

❑❑ **What medication overdose can cause a patient to present with tinnitus?**

Aspirin.

❑❑ **What is capillary refill time?**

The amount of time required for color to return to the nail beds after application of slight pressure which caused blanching.

❑❑ **What is the emergency treatment for a corneal injury from a caustic substance?**

Flush both eyes with copious amounts of water for 20-30 minutes.

❑❑ **How do you remove a patient's artificial eye?**

Depress the lower lid.

❑❑ **How do you clean an artificial eye?**

Soap and water.

❑❑ **What does severe pain after cataract surgery indicate?**

Bleeding in the eye.

❑❑ **What does the term "ascites" mean?**

An accumulation of fluid in the peritoneal cavity.

❑❑ **What parts of the skin are affected in a partial thickness burn?**

The epidermis and dermis.

❑❑ **What is the difference between an axillary temperature and an oral temperature?**

An axillary temp is one degree Fahrenheit lower than an oral temp.

❑❑ **What does the term "P.C." mean?**

Take after meals.

❑❑ **What does the term "gauge" refer to?**

The inside diameter of a needle. The smaller the gauge the larger the diameter.

❒❒ **How many permanent teeth do adults normally have?**

32.

❒❒ **What type of insulin can be mixed with other types of insulin?**

Regular insulin.

❒❒ **What 4 things should you assess when measuring a patient's pulse?**

Rate, rhythm, quality, and strength of the pulse.

❒❒ **Describe decorticate posturing.**

The patient's arms are adducted and flexed, with the wrists and fingers flexed on the chest. The legs are extended and internally rotated with plantar flexion of the feet.

❒❒ **Define retroflexion.**

An abnormal backward tilt of an organ that has folded over on itself.

❒❒ **Define rhonchi.**

Abnormal breath sounds caused by obstruction with thick secretions, muscular spasm, neoplasm or external pressure.

❒❒ **What factors are measured by the Glasgow Coma Scale?**

Verbal, eye, and motor response.

❒❒ **For what are thrombocytopenic patients at risk?**

Life-threatening internal and external hemorrhages.

❒❒ **How long does it take for a synthetic cast to reach its maximum strength?**

30 minutes.

❒❒ **How long does it take for a plaster cast to reach its maximum strength?**

48 hours.

❒❒ **What are the indications of circulatory interference?**

Pallor or redness, cyanosis, coolness, numbness, and decreased capillary refill.

❒❒ **What is indicated by a rising pulse rate and falling blood pressure in a postoperative patient?**

Hemorrhage and impending shock.

❒❒ **How long should a patient's identification bracelet remain in place?**

Until he/she has been discharged from the hospital.

❒❒ **If an IV was inserted during an emergency and/or outside the hospital, how soon should it be changed?**

Within 24 hours.

❒❒ **What temperature should shower and bath water not exceed?**

105 degrees Fahrenheit (40.5 degrees Celsius).

❒❒ **What is the major complication of Bell's palsy?**

Corneal inflammation (keratitis).

❒❒ **What type of footwear should be used by patients who are recovering from a CVA?**

High top sneakers (to prevent foot drop and contractures).

❒❒ **What is the most common complication of a hip fracture?**

Thromboembolism.

❒❒ **How should a patient climb stairs when using crutches?**

Lead with the uninvolved leg, and follow with the crutches and involved leg.

❒❒ **How does a patient descend stairs when using crutches?**

Lead with the crutches and the involved leg, and follow with the uninvolved leg.

❒❒ **What are the symptoms of Meniere's disease?**

Vertigo, tinnitus, and hearing loss.

❒❒ **What is the treatment for mild to moderate varicose veins?**

Antiembolism stockings and moderate walking, which will minimize venous pooling.

❒❒ **What does the term "gynecomastia" refer to?**

Excessive mammary gland development and increased breast size in boys and men.

❒❒ **What findings are observed in the early stages of Alzheimer's disease?**

Inappropriate affect, disorientation to time, paranoia, memory loss, and an impaired judgement.

❒❒ **When should a physician sign verbal and telephone orders?**

Within 24 hours.

❑❑ **What is the most common symptom of osteoarthritis?**

Joint pain that is relieved by rest.

❑❑ **What is the normal daily urine volume of an adult?**

1,200-1,500 ml/day.

❑❑ **When administering a nitroprusside sodium IV, what special care should be taken with the medication bag?**

Wrap the IV bag in foil to shield it from light.

❑❑ **T/F: The patient should not be involved in planning her/his own pain management.**

False.

❑❑ **What group of antibiotics must be used with caution in penicillin-allergic patients?**

Cephalosporins.

❑❑ **How long should a patient fast before having a plasma glucose test?**

12-14 hours.

❑❑ **What are the alterable risk factors for coronary artery disease?**

High cholesterol and/or triglyceride levels, diabetes, hypertension, and cigarette smoking.

❑❑ **What are the major complications of an acute myocardial infarction?**

Thromboembolism, cardiogenic shock, left ventricular rupture, acute heart failure, and arrhythmias.

❑❑ **What is the treatment of choice for patients with pulseless ventricular tachycardia?**

Defibrillation.

❑❑ **What does the term "ataxia" mean?**

An impaired ability to coordinate movement.

❑❑ **What is the most common vascular complication found in patients with diabetes mellitus?**

Atherosclerosis.

❑❑ **When assessing a patient's heart, where is the point of maximal impulse usually found?**

Fifth intercostal space, left mid-clavicular line.

❑❑ **What is the cause of an S1 sound heard on auscultation?**

Closure of the mitral and tricuspid valves.

❑❑ **What is the most common nosocomial infection?**

Urinary tract infection.

❑❑ **What are the 2 most important nutrients for proper wound healing?**

Vitamin C and protein.

❑❑ **What are the symptoms of Grave's disease?**

Nervousness, weight loss, sweating, diarrhea, heat intolerance, an enlarged thyroid, tremors, and palpitations.

❑❑ **Describe the symptoms of the last stage of Alzheimer's disease.**

Blank facial expression, seizures, loss of appetite, emaciation, irritability, and total dependence.

❑❑ **What is the purpose of Buck's traction?**

To immobilize and reduce the spasms in a fractured hip.

❑❑ **How often should you assess the neurocirculatory status in a patient with a fractured hip?**

Every 2 hours.

❑❑ **What is the major circulatory complication of an immobilized patient?**

Pulmonary embolism.

❑❑ **What should be your top nursing priority in caring for a terminally ill patient who is near death?**

Comfort.

❑❑ **What is the laxative of choice for patients recovering from rectal surgery, postpartum constipation, or acute myocardial infarction?**

Docusate sodium (Colace).

❑❑ **In a hospitalized alcoholic, when do DT's most commonly occur?**

3-4 days after admission.

❑❑ **At what level of unconjugated bilirubin can brainstem dysfunction occur?**

20-25 mg/dl.

❑❑ **What are the classic symptoms of diabetes mellitus?**

Polyphagia, weight loss, polydipsia, and polyuria.

❑❑ **How do rapid-acting and long-acting insulin preparations differ in their appearance?**

Rapid-acting insulins are clear, while long-acting insulins are cloudy.

❑❑ **What is the best time to check a patient's glucose?**

Before each meal and at bedtime.

❑❑ **How long does it take for long-acting insulin to act?**

4-8 hours.

❑❑ **What are some conditions that cause an increase in insulin requirement?**

Growth, increased food intake, multiple medications, illness, infection, stress, surgery, and pregnancy.

❑❑ **What is the definition of an insulin-resistant patient?**

A patient who requires more than 200 units of insulin each day.

❑❑ **What are the signs and symptoms of hypoglycemia?**

Tachycardia, palpitations, tremors, pallor, and sweating.

❑❑ **What medication should be given to a patient who is hypoglycemic and unconscious?**

An IM injection of glucagon.

❑❑ **What are the findings in a patient with diabetic ketoacidosis?**

Polyuria, polydipsia, anorexia, muscle cramps and vomiting, Kussmaul's respirations, stupor, and coma.

❑❑ **What are the signs and symptoms of myxedema coma?**

Lethargy, stupor, decreased level of consciousness, delayed deep tendon reflexes, progressive respiratory depression, weight gain, hypoglycemia, dry skin and hair, and hypothermia.

❑❑ **What are the signs and symptoms of colorectal cancer?**

Rectal bleeding, abdominal pain, anorexia, weight loss, anemia, malaise, changes in bowel habits, and constipation or diarrhea.

❑❑ **CAUTION is used to express the 7 warning signs of cancer. What does this abbreviation mean?**

Change in bowel or bladder habits.
A sore that does not heal.
Unusual bleeding or drainage.

Thickening or lump in the breast or elsewhere.
Indigestion or difficulty swallowing.
Obvious change in a wart or mole.
Nagging cough or hoarseness.

❑❑ **T/F: Unlimited visitors are allowed when your patient is under going sealed internal radiation.**

False.

❑❑ **What causes shortening of the trunk in an elderly person?**

The loss of bone mass.

❑❑ **Define kyphosis.**

Spinal curvature, commonly known as humpback.

❑❑ **What are the common pathologic conditions of the musculoskelatal system in the elderly?**

Arthritis, osteoarthritis, gout, and fractures.

❑❑ **What are the sites most effected by osteoporosis?**

The vertebrae, hips, and the wrists.

❑❑ **What causes kyphosis in elderly women?**

The collapse of fractures of the thoracic vertebra.

❑❑ **What are some of the risk factors associated with osteoporosis?**

Smoking, high caffeine intake, excessive alcohol intake, and a history of low dietary calcium intake.

❑❑ **T/F: After menopause, bone loss decreases.**

True.

MATERNAL-INFANT PEARLS

"Decide promptly, but never give your reasons.
Your decision may be right,
but your reasons are sure to be wrong."
Lord Mansfield

❑❑ **What nursing measures can be suggested for the treatment of hemorrhoids?**

A high fiber diet, sitz baths, and good hygiene.

❑❑ **How is fetal lung maturity assessed?**

By measuring the ratio of lecithin to sphingomyelin (L/S). An L/S ratio greater than 2 and the presence of phosphatidyl glycerol verifies that the fetal lungs are mature.

❑❑ **What drug can be given to a mother to avoid respiratory distress syndrome in her unborn infant?**

If the fetus is > 32 weeks, betamethasone can be administered 48–72 hours before delivery to augment surfactant production.

❑❑ **What is a Bartholin's cyst?**

An obstructed Bartholin's duct that results in an abscess.

❑❑ **What bone is most commonly fractured in newborns?**

The clavicle. Treat by pinning the infant's sleeve to the front of her shirt.

❑❑ **You are examining a newborn baby who has kidney-shaped soles of his feet and a medial deviation of his heels. You are not able to dorsiflex his feet. What is the diagnosis?**

"Club foot," which is medically known as talipes equinovarus. Mild cases may be attributed to in utero positioning. More serious cases are due to anatomical abnormalities, such as congenital convex pes valgus or spina bifida.

❑❑ **Is constipation more common in breast-fed or formula fed infants?**

Formula fed. It is very rare in breast-fed infants. Treatment involves increasing the amount of fluid and/or sugar in the formula and adding prune juice, fruits, cereal, and vegetables to the baby's diet to increase bulk.

❑❑ **When is the risk of congenital defects from maternal rubella infection greatest?**

In the first few months of gestation. During months 1–3, there is a 30–60% risk of congenital defects. By the fourth month, the risk is only 10%. By 5–9 months, the chances that the child has a defect are rare.

❒❒ **When are women at their greatest risk for psychiatric illness?**

During the first few weeks post partum. It most often occurs in patients who are primiparous, have poor social support, or have a history of depression.

❒❒ **When does post partum psychosis begin?**

Within the first week to 10 days following childbirth. A second, smaller peak occurs 6–8 weeks post partum. This second peak correlates with the first post partum menses. The risk of psychosis is lowest during pregnancy.

❒❒ **What percentage of pregnancies result in spontaneous abortions?**

20–25%.

❒❒ **What is the most common cause of spontaneous abortions?**

Chromosomal abnormality.

❒❒ **How does a spontaneous abortion most commonly present?**

Pain followed by bleeding.

❒❒ **Before what gestational age do most spontaneous abortions occur?**

8–9 weeks.

❒❒ **Define the term "missed abortion."**

There is no uterine growth, no cervical dilation, no passage of fetal tissue, and minimal cramping or bleeding. Diagnosis is made by the absence of fetal heart tones and an empty gestational sac on ultrasound.

❒❒ **What are the risk factors for abruptio placentae?**

Smoking, hypertension, multiparity, trauma, and previous abruptio placenta.

❒❒ **What are the presenting signs and symptoms of abruptio placentae?**

Placental separation before delivery is associated with vaginal bleeding (78%), abdominal pain (66%), as well as tetanic uterine contractions, uterine irritability, and fetal death.

❒❒ **What common non-gynecologic condition presents with lower abdominal pain?**

Appendicitis.

❒❒ **At what gestational age is amniocentesis performed?**

16–18 weeks .

❒❒ **How soon after implantation can ß-hCG be detected?**

2–3 days.

❒❒ **ß-hCG levels rise at what rate?**

They double every 48 hours.

❒❒ **What is the most common benign breast tumor?**

Fibroadenomas. They are most common in women under 30. They are usually solitary, mobile masses with distinct borders.

❒❒ **What medicines are contraindicated in breast-feeding mothers?**

Tetracycline, warfarin, and chloramphenicol.

❒❒ **What is the most common cancer in women?**

Lung cancer. Breast Cancer is second; colorectal cancer is third.

❒❒ **What are the American Cancer Society's 1996 recommendations for mammography?**

Every 1–2 years after age 40, annually after age 50.

❒❒ **What are the risk factors for breast cancer, and how do they compare with the risk factors for endometrial cancer?**

Risk factors for both cancers include nulliparity, early menarche, late menopause, significant amounts of unopposed estrogen, and prior ovarian, endometrial, or breast cancer. Unopposed estrogen is a much greater risk in endometrial cancer than in breast cancer. Risk factors specific to breast cancer include family history, age over 40, high fat intake, radiation of the breast, or cellular atypia in fibrocystic disease.

❒❒ **What is Peau d'orange?**

Peau d'orange, French for "skin of the orange," is the dimpling and thickening of the breast in patients who have breast cancer. It is caused by an obstruction of the lymphatics and a local invasion of the tumor, which pulls on the Cooper's ligaments and, in turn, pulls on the skin.

❒❒ **What is the American Cancer Society's 1996 recommendation for PAP smears?**

Annually for 3 years, starting at age 18 or when the patient becomes sexually active, then every 1–3 years thereafter.

❒❒ **How long after the removal of Norplant capsules can patients become pregnant?**

Ovulation usually occurs within 3 months.

❒❒ **In which patients are oral contraceptives contraindicated?**

Patients with DVT's, MI's, history of smoking, liver tumors, breast cancer or other estrogen-dependent tumors, heart disease, vascular disease, or a prior thromboembolism.

❒❒ **What are the risk factors for ectopic pregnancy?**

Prior scarring of the fallopian tubes from infection (i.e., PID or salpingitis), IUD's, previous ectopic pregnancy, tubal ligation, and STD's.

❒❒ **When does an ectopic pregnancy most commonly present?**

6–8 weeks. Patients usually present with amenorrhea and sharp abdominal or pelvic pain. A mass can be felt in half of these patients. ß-hCG confirms pregnancy, and an ultrasound will generally confirm an ectopic pregnancy.

❒❒ **What is the risk of a repeat ectopic pregnancy?**

10–15%.

❒❒ **When can an abdominal ultrasound find an intrauterine gestational sac?**

In the fifth week. The fetal pole is found in the sixth week, and an embryonic mass with cardiac motion can be detected by the seventh week.

❒❒ **At what point does magnesium sulfate become toxic?**

Loss of reflexes occurs at levels > 8 mEq/l, and respiratory arrest occurs at levels > 12 mEq/l.

❒❒ **Which 2 drugs are used to treat eclampsia?**

Magnesium sulfate 4–6 g IV bolus, followed by a 2 g/h infusion; and hydralazine, 10–20 mg IV. Labetalol may also be used.

❒❒ **How much blood does a standard size pad absorb?**

20–30 ml.

❒❒ **Is the hCG level high or low in a molar pregnancy?**

High.

❒❒ **How can lung maturity be assessed in the fetus?**

The L/S ratio. If the ratio of lecithin to sphingomyelin is over 2, then the fetal lungs are mature.

❒❒ **A couple is having trouble conceiving. You tell them to keep track of the wife's temperature. When should they have intercourse?**

Ovulation causes a 0.4°F rise in a woman's basal body temperature. Therefore, when the woman's temperature peaks, it is the best time to try to conceive.

❒❒ **A breast-feeding mother is complaining of fever, chills, and a swollen red breast. What is the most likely causative organism?**

Staphylococcus aureus is the most common cause of mastitis. Mastitis is seldom present in the first week post partum. It is most often seen 3–4 weeks post partum.

❑❑ **Match the following terms with the appropriate definitions.**

1) Menorrhagia	a) Bleeding between menstrual periods
2) Metrorrhagia (hypermenorrhea)	b) Excessive amount of blood or duration
3) Menometrorrhagia	c) Excessive amount of blood at irregular frequencies

Answers: 1) b, 2) a, 3) c.

❑❑ **Match the following menstrual terms to their definitions.**

1) Hypermenorrhea	a) Menstrual periods > 35 days apart
2) Oligomenorrhea	b) Menstrual periods < 21 days apart
3) Polymenorrhea	c) Menorrhagia

Answers: 1) c, 2) a, 3) b.

❑❑ **The ovarian luteal phase corresponds to what phase of the uterus?**

The secretory phase. The luteal phase begins after ovulation. At this time, the expelled follicle is called the corpus luteum. The corpus luteum secretes estradiol and progesterone, which cause secretory ducts to develop in the endometrial lining.

❑❑ **Morning sickness is due to increased levels of what?**

ß-hCG.

❑❑ **T/F: A woman with pelvic inflammatory disease (PID) is most likely to have an exacerbation of symptoms when she menstruates?**

True. The breakdown of the cervical mucus antibacterial barrier allows bacteria to ascend from the lower tract to the upper tract. Pelvic exam, intercourse, and exercise can all exacerbate symptoms.

❑❑ **What 2 organisms cause most cases of PID?**

Neisseria gonorrhea and Chlamydia trachomatis.

❑❑ **What are the risk factors for placenta previa?**

Previous cesarean section, previous placenta previa, multiparity, multiple induced abortions, and multiple gestations.

❑❑ **During what week of gestation does a mother begin to feel fetal movement?**

The sixteenth to twentieth week.

❑❑ **By what week of gestation can a doppler detect fetal heart tones?**

The twelfth week.

❑❑ **By what week of gestation can ultrasound detect an intrauterine fetal pole?**

Sixth to seventh week.

❑❑ **During pregnancy, a woman's blood volume will increase by what percent?**

45%. To compensate, her heart rate will increase 10–15 bpm.

❑❑ **T/F: A systolic murmur can be heard in most pregnant women.**

True. 90% of all pregnant women will have a systolic murmur on exam.

❑❑ **What is the average weight gain of the mother during a single pregnancy?**

25–30 lbs.

❑❑ **Why should pregnant women rest in the lateral decubitus position?**

To avert supine hypotension syndrome caused by compression of the inferior rena cava on the uterus.

❑❑ **What vaccines are contraindicated in the pregnant patient?**

Smallpox, measles, mumps, rubella, and varicella.

❑❑ **Teenage pregnancies are associated with increased risks of what complications?**

Gonorrhea, syphilis, toxemia, anemia, malnutrition, low birth weight babies, and perinatal mortality.

❑❑ **Define pregnancy-induced hypertension.**

An increase in the systolic pressure > 30 mm Hg, or an increase in diastolic pressure > 15 mm Hg over base line, measured on 2 separate occasions at least 6 hours apart.

❑❑ **Define preeclampsia.**

HTN (a systolic pressure > 160 mm Hg or a diastolic pressure > 110 mm Hg) after 20 weeks EGA, with generalized edema or proteinuria of 5 gm or more during a 24 hour period.

❑❑ **Define eclampsia.**

Preeclampsia, plus grand mal seizures or coma.

❑❑ **When can the seizures of eclampsia occur?**

Before, during, and after labor.

❑❑ **What factors cause a women to be more likely to have preeclampsia?**

Preeclampsia occurs most commonly in primiparous women. Older women, and women with multiple gestations, hypertensive disease, or prior vascular disease are also at risk.

❑❑ **How long should treatment continue after delivery in a woman with preeclampsia?**

24 hours. The cure of preeclampsia is delivery. Antihypertensives and antiseizure medication (IV magnesium) should be continued until there is no longer a risk to the mother.

❑❑ **Why is Rh status important in a pregnant patient?**

If the mother is Rh negative and the fetus is Rh positive, fetal anemia, hydrops, and fetal loss can result. Rh immunoglobulin should be given to all Rh negative patients.

❑❑ **When should RhoGAM be given to the Rh negative mother?**

At 28 weeks or whenever bleeding occurs (e.g., amniocentesis or trauma).

❑❑ **What predisposes a woman to yeast infections?**

Diabetes, oral contraceptives, and antibiotics.

❑❑ **What is the most common cause of vaginitis?**

Candida albicans.

❑❑ **What is the treatment for gonorrhea?**

Ceftriaxone and doxycycline. The latter is given because half of all patients infected with gonorrhea are simultaneously infected with chlamydia.

❑❑ **What causes toxic shock syndrome (TSS)?**

An exotoxin composed of certain strains of Staphylococcus aureus. Other organisms causing toxic shock syndrome include: Group A Streptococcus, Pseudomonas aeruginosa, and Streptococcus pneumoniae. Tampons, IUDs, septic abortions, sponges, soft tissue abscesses, osteomyelitis, nasal packing, and post partum infections can also house these organisms.

❑❑ **The average gestational period for a single birth is 39 weeks. What is the average gestational period for twins?**

35 weeks. Prematurity is a large risk factor of respiratory distress syndrome. One half of all perinatal deaths involving twins are due to respiratory distress syndrome.

❑❑ **What is the most common type of urinary fistula?**

Vesicovaginal fistulas. They most commonly occur after surgical procedures, but they can also occur with invasive cervical carcinoma or radiotherapy due to cervical cancer.

❑❑ **Venereal warts are caused by what virus?**

Human papilloma virus types 6 and 11.

❑❑ **What fetal heart rates are considered normal?**

120–160 bpm. If bradycardia is detected, position the mother on her left side, give oxygen and an IV fluid bolus.

❑❑ **What causes variable decelerations?**

Transient umbilical cord compression, which often change with maternal position.

❑❑ **What anticoagulant should be used on pregnant patients?**

Heparin, as it does not cross the placenta.

❑❑ **What antiemetic agents should be used in pregnant patients?**

Prochlorperazine (Compazine) or trimethobenzamide (Tigan).

❑❑ **What are the 3 types of breech presentation?**

Frank breech: thighs flexed, legs extended.
Complete breech: at least one leg flexed.
Incomplete breech/footling breech: at least 1 foot below the buttocks with both thighs extended.

❑❑ **What is the most common breech position?**

Frank breech.

❑❑ **What percentage of women can have vaginal births after having a low transverse c-section?**

75%.

❑❑ **What are the 4 stages of labor and delivery?**

First stage: onset of labor to complete dilation of the cervix.
Second stage: cervical dilation to birth.
Third stage: birth to delivery of the placenta.
Fourth stage: placenta delivery to stability of the mother (about 6 hours).

❑❑ **What is the difference between a classic c-section and a newer c-section?**

A classic c-section is done with a vertical incision in the uterus. This type of c-section predisposes women to future uterine rupture. Hence, subsequent deliveries should be made via c-section as well. The newer c-sections are done with low transverse incisions; they have a much lower rate of uterine rupture with subsequent deliveries.

❑❑ **What are the 6 movements of delivery?**

1) Descent
2) Flexion
3) Internal rotation
4) Extension
5) External rotation
6) Expulsion

❑❑ **A patient who is 3 days post partum has foul lochia and a tender, boggy uterus. What is the diagnosis?**

Endometritis. This typically occurs 1–3 days post partum.

❑❑ **What is the most common cause of a prolonged active phase of labor?**

Cephalopelvic disproportion. Contraction of a narrowed midpelvis is the most common cause of cephalopelvic disproportion.

❑❑ **What is the most common cause of post partum hemorrhage?**

Uterine atony.

❑❑ **What practice is routinely done to decrease the risk of post partum hemorrhage?**

Uterine massage and oxytocin.

❑❑ **What is the number one cause of maternal mortality?**

Thromboembolism. The risk progressively increases throughout pregnancy, peaking during the post partum period at > 5 times the non-pregnant rate. Other causes of maternal mortality include hemorrhage, infection, and hypertension.

❑❑ **How can ruptured membranes be diagnosed?**

Nitrazine paper turns blue and a fern shaped pattern is seen under the microscope in the presence of amniotic fluid.

❑❑ **What is the most common medical complication of pregnancy?**

Urinary tract infections.

❑❑ **Is preeclampsia more common in primagravidas or multigravidas?**

Primagravidas.

❑❑ **Name 6 risk factors for ectopic pregnancy.**

1) Advanced maternal age
2) PID
3) Prior ectopic pregnancy
4) History of pelvic surgery or tubal ligation
5) IUD
6) In vitro fertilization

❑❑ **At what age can routine pap smears be discontinued?**

By age 70 if the patient has had several negative exams. Cervical cancer reaches a plateau at this point, so further screening is not necessary.

❑❑ **Should pregnant women abstain from intercourse?**

No. There is no risk to mother or fetus if mother engages in sex with one orgasm in the first 2 trimesters.

In the third trimester, anorgasmic intercourse is safe until the 34th week. Intercourse should be avoided if there is bleeding.

❒❒ **What routine screenings should be performed on all pregnant women?**

Hepatitis B, syphilis, rubella, gonorrhea, and other STDs. Women at high risk for HIV should also be screened for this disease.

❒❒ **When should RhoGAM be used?**

RhoGAM (anti-Rh immunoglobulin) should be used within 3 days of the birth of a child with Rh+ blood if the mother is Rh-. It should also be used in the event of any mixing of fetal and maternal blood (e.g., trauma). RhoGAM is safe because it does not pass the placenta barrier.

❒❒ **Why does estrogen protect against coronary artery disease?**

Estrogen decreases the amount of cholesterol, LDLs, and VLDLs, while it increases HDLs.

❒❒ **What gynecological infection presents with a malodorous, itchy, white to grayish, and sometimes frothy vaginal discharge?**

Trichomoniasis.

❒❒ **Describe the presentation of placenta previa.**

Painless, bright red vaginal bleeding.

❒❒ **Describe the presentation of abruptio placentae.**

Painful, dark red vaginal bleeding.

❒❒ **What is the most common cause of immediate post partum hemorrhage?**

Uterine atony, followed by vaginal/cervical lacerations and retained placenta or placental fragments.

❒❒ **Newborns should stop losing weight how many days after birth?**

About 6 days.

❒❒ **Projectile vomiting in the neonate is often associated with pyloric stenosis. When this is the case, such vomiting becomes a prominent sign at what age?**

2–3 weeks.

❒❒ **What is the most frequent sign of an ectopic pregnancy?**

Abdominal pain. Amenorrhea is the second most common sign.

❒❒ **What WBC count is expected during pregnancy?**

WBC counts of 15,000–20,000 are considered normal during pregnancy.

❏❏ When monitoring a pregnant trauma victim, are the vital signs of the mother or the fetus most sensitive?

The fetus. This is because the fetal heart rate is more sensitive to inadequate resuscitation. Remember that the mother may lose 10–20% of her blood volume without a change in vital signs, whereas the baby's heart rate may increase or decrease above 160 or below 120, indicating significant fetal distress. The most common pitfall is failure to adequately resuscitate the mother.

❏❏ What 2 findings on physical exam indicate uterine rupture?

Loss of uterine contour and palpable fetal part.

❏❏ What physical exam findings may be discovered in abruptio placenta?

Rapidly increasing fundal height secondary to bleeding into the uterus, or a higher than expected fundal height.

❏❏ What is the number one risk factor for uterine rupture?

Previous cesarean section.

❏❏ A young patient has a threatened abortion in the first trimester. Laboratory studies reveal she is Rh negative and her husband is Rh positive. Is RhoGAM indicated?

Yes.

❏❏ What are the signs and symptoms of preeclampsia?

Upper abdominal pain, headache, visual complaints, cardiac decompensation, creatinine greater than 2, proteinuria greater than 100 mg per deciliter, and a blood pressure of greater than 160 mm Hg systolic or 110 mm Hg diastolic. Preeclampsia is most common in nulliparous women late in pregnancy, typically after 20 weeks gestation. Also look for edema, hypertension, and proteinuria.

❏❏ In which trimester of pregnancy is UTI and pyelonephritis most common?

Third.

❏❏ Describe the presentation of a patient with Gardnerella vaginitis.

On physical exam, a frothy, grayish-white, fishy smelling vaginal discharge is present.

❏❏ What effect does pregnancy have on BUN and creatinine?

Both are decreased. This is the result of increased renal blood flow and increased glomerular filtration rate.

❏❏ When can one auscultate the fetal heart?

Ultrasound: 6 weeks
Doppler: 10–12 weeks
Stethoscope: 18–20 weeks

❒❒ What is the normal blood pressure in a newborn?

60 mmHg.

❒❒ If a pregnant patient is choking, what modification should you make when performing the standard Heimlich maneuver?

Use a chest thrust (instead of an abdominal one) to decrease potential harm to the fetus.

❒❒ What assessment should be a high priority after a patient has received an epidural?

Blood pressure. An epidural can cause hypotension, because it blocks the autonomic nervous system.

❒❒ What instructions should you give to a patient with recurring bouts of vaginitis?

Wear loose fitting clothing, perform good hygiene (especially after elimination), and avoid non-cotton undergarments.

❒❒ You notice that a newborn's eyes appear crossed, yet the physician is not concerned. Why?

It is not uncommon for a newborn's eyes to be temporarily crossed due to the immature neuromuscular control of the eye muscles.

❒❒ What is the best method to use when teaching infant care to a patient?

Hands-on-training and return demonstrations of the techniques learned.

❒❒ T/F: A pregnant, insulin-dependent diabetic is at risk for sudden hypoglycemia.

True. Insulin needs and metabolism are affected by pregnancy, making sudden hypoglycemic episodes more common for diabetics.

❒❒ What should you teach a pregnant, insulin dependent diabetic concerning exercise?

Exercise is important, but should always be done with family or friends because of the increased chance for sudden hypoglycemic episodes.

❒❒ What does a positive Homan's sign indicate?

The possibility that thrombophlebitis or a deep venous thrombosis is present in the lower extremities.

❒❒ How do you assess for Homan's sign?

Ask the patient to stretch her legs out with the knee slightly flexed while you dorsiflex the foot. A positive sign is present when pain is felt at the back of the knee or calf.

❒❒ What complications can result from heparin therapy during pregnancy?

Preterm labor and maternal hemorrhage.

❒❒ A patient at 36 weeks gestation has leg edema, a headache, and an elevated blood pressure.

What is the most likely cause of these symptoms?

Pregnancy induced hypertension (PIH).

❑❑ **What is the common intravenous medication used to treat PIH?**

IV Magnesium Sulfate.

❑❑ **Is it normal for a patient on magnesium sulfate therapy to feel tired?**

Yes. Magnesium sulfate acts as a central nervous system depressant and often makes the patient drowsy.

❑❑ **A newborn's respiratory rate is 50 breaths per minute and is shallow with periods of apnea that last up to 5 seconds. What should you do?**

Just continue to monitor the newborn, as this is a normal respiratory pattern.

❑❑ **Pregnant patients are told to avoid undercooked meats and avoid scooping the cat's litter box for what reason?**

To prevent a toxoplasmosis infection.

❑❑ **What is a good indicator of fetal lung maturity in a pregnant diabetic?**

The presence of phosphatidyglycerol in the amniotic fluid.

❑❑ **During pregnancy, the woman's caloric needs increase by how much per day?**

300 calories.

❑❑ **What is the best method for relieving constipation in pregnant patients?**

Increase fluid intake and add more fiber to the diet. Medications should be avoided unless approved by the physician.

❑❑ **Why is back pain a common complaint during pregnancy?**

The growing fetus causes the woman to develop a swayback, which acts as a counterbalance. This causes stress on the back muscles and, therefore, increases discomfort.

❑❑ **Other than medication, is there a remedy for back pain in the third trimester?**

The pelvic tilt exercise is often helpful.

❑❑ **What is the primary reason for turning a patient turn every 2 hours after general anesthesia?**

To prevent pulmonary complications such as atelectasis, which could lead to infection.

❑❑ **What week does the heart begin to beat in the embryo?**

Between the third and fourth week.

❑❑ **What are Kegel exercises?**

Tightening and releasing of the pubococcygeus muscle.

❑❑ **Why are Kegel exercises important during pregnancy?**

They increase elasticity of the pubococcygeus muscle, increasing its tone and preventing future bladder and uterine problems.

❑❑ **When is medication used to control a first trimester patient's nausea?**

When the benefits of drug therapy outweigh the risks to the mother or fetus.

❑❑ **A patient in her 6th month of pregnancy complains of feeling dizzy, short of breath, and clammy when lying on her back for long periods of time. What is the most likely cause?**

Supine hypotension.

❑❑ **What is the cause of supine hypotension during pregnancy?**

The weight of the uterus compresses the inferior vena cava, decreasing the return of blood to the heart, thus decreasing cardiac output, which lowers the blood pressure.

❑❑ **What is the most objective sign of pregnancy you can assess?**

Fetal movement felt by the examiner.

❑❑ **A patient in her 36th week of pregnancy presents with vaginal bleeding. What should be your first assessment?**

Assess the mother's blood pressure and the fetal heart tones to determine the condition of the mother and fetus.

❑❑ **What is the most common complication found in pregnant adolescents?**

Pregnancy induced hypertension.

❑❑ **What methods can be used to determine the nutritional status of a pregnant patient?**

Weight, body measurements, fetal measurements, and a 24 hour history of food intake.

❑❑ **How does smoking during pregnancy affect the fetus?**

Lowers birth weight and develops a smaller than normal brain.

❑❑ **In which trimester of pregnancy do women generally feel their best?**

The second.

❑❑ **What emotions and fears are usually felt during the third trimester?**

Feelings of "ugliness," alterations in body self image, and anxiety about the coming labor and delivery.

❒❒ The vitals of a postpartum patient are: BP 150/100, pulse 72, resp 22, and temp 99.0 F. The doctor has ordered Methergine 0.2 mg PO. What is your best response?

Do not give the drug. The patient is hypertensive and Methergine can worsen this symptom.

❒❒ What is the effect of giving methylergonovine (Methergine) to a pregnant patient?

It causes the uterus to contract after delivery so that bleeding will be lessened in the postpartum recovery period.

❒❒ T/F: Pregnancy in the adolescent patient usually results in greater dependence on the patient's parents.

True.

❒❒ What effect can prolonged pregnancy-induced hypertension (PIH) have on the fetus?

PIH reduces blood flow to the placenta, which can result in intrauterine growth retardation, and a decrease in the ability of the fetus to handle the stress of labor.

❒❒ What is a biophysical profile?

A test conducted on the fetus in utero that gives an indication of fetal well-being.

❒❒ What characteristics are measured in a biophysical profile?

Fetal breathing movements, fetal body movements, tone, amniotic fluid volume, and fetal heart rate activity.

❒❒ What effect does cocaine have on labor and the fetus?

Preterm labor, increased uterine contractions, intrauterine growth retardation, and the potential for a sick, addicted infant.

❒❒ A pregnant patient with a known history of crack cocaine use is in labor. How should you prepare for the delivery?

Be prepared for a precipitous labor and notify the neonatalogist of the infant's high risk status.

❒❒ You assess a patient 24 hours after delivery and note a large amount of lochia rubra with many clots. The patient has used 15 pads in the past 8 hours. Should the M.D. be notified?

Yes. This bleeding is above average (8-19 pads per 24 hour period is normal).

❒❒ After lochia rubra, what terms are used to describe the next phases of postpartum discharge?

Lochia serosa, followed by lochia alba.

❒❒ A patient who is in her eighth week of pregnancy calls and says she is experiencing a slight amount of vaginal bleeding. How should you instruct this patient?

The patient should come is as soon as possible, and she should save any pads or discharge. Further evaluation is needed to determine if this is a threatened abortion.

❑❑ **Why does a lack of surfactant cause respiratory distress in the premature newborn?**

Surfactant increases lung compliance and decreases the amount of inspiratory pressure needed to breathe. Without it, the lung's capacity is greatly reduced.

❑❑ **What should you look for when assessing for post delivery uterine hemorrhage?**

Amount and quality of lochia, early signs and symptoms of shock, fundal tone, and vital signs.

❑❑ **What is the preferred position for the administration of an epidural?**

Lateral left with legs flexed and back curved so that the arms are "hugging" the knees.

❑❑ **The fetal monitor reveals a slowing of the fetal heart rate during each contraction. What simple nursing measure can be done to help relieve fetal distress?**

Have the patient lie on her left side.

❑❑ **What is the purpose of the above measure?**

It increases blood flow to the uterus by relieving pressure on the vena cava.

❑❑ **What would be an indication that too many visitors are in the room while a patient is in labor?**

If she is unable to focus on her breathing techniques because of all the distractions in the room, then some of the visitors should be removed.

❑❑ **A patient complains of a "fluttering" sensation in her chest. She is taking terbutaline (Brethine) SQ for premature contractions. Should you notify the M.D.?**

No. This is a common side effect of terbutaline (Brethine) and it can be ignored unless the vital signs indicate distress.

❑❑ **What drug is commonly ordered to counteract the effect of terbutaline (Brethine)?**

Hydroxyzine hydrochloride (Vistaril).

❑❑ **What is the Ferguson reflex?**

An uncontrollable urge to bear down during labor, which is caused by the presenting part approaching or touching the perineal floor.

❑❑ **In what stage of labor does a patient have the uncontrollable desire to push?**

Stage II.

❑❑ **What are the early signs that indicate the fetus is in distress during labor?**

The fetus is extremely active and tachycardic.

❑❑ **T/F: A pregnant teenager often has problems with low self esteem, indecision, poor self image, accountability, and egocentrism.**

True.

❑❑ **What percentage of weight is normal for a newborn to lose in the first few days after birth?**

5 - 10%.

❑❑ **A patient in her first trimester complains of an increase in a clear vaginal discharge. What should be your first action?**

Explain that an increase in vaginal discharge is normal during pregnancy unless redness, itching or foul odor are present.

❑❑ **What should you say to a patient who wishes to douche during her pregnancy?**

Don't! Douching is contraindicated in pregnancy. Daily washing of the perineal area with soap and water should be sufficient.

❑❑ **A patient receiving magnesium sulfate for 3 hours to treat PIH has a BP of 160/100, DTR of +1, pulse of 100, a respiratory rate of 9, and urine output of 15 cc/hr. How much longer should you continue the infusion?**

Stop the infusion now. The patient is beginning to show signs of toxicity.

❑❑ **What assessment data from the above patient indicated that toxicity from magnesium sulfate could be beginning?**

The DTR's should be +2 and urine output 25-30cc/hr. Other symptoms would be flushing of the skin and the complaint of feeling warm.

❑❑ **A patient in Stage I of labor has mild contractions, appears anxious, and is requesting pain medication. What should you do?**

First, try to find the source of her anxiety and work on helping her relieve it. Medication, if given too early, can prolong labor.

❑❑ **A patient is found crying 3 days after her emergency c-section. She states that she feels like a failure. What is she most likely grieving over?**

The loss of her anticipated normal birth experience. This is normal for many women who have an unplanned c-section.

❑❑ **What effect can a pudendal block have on labor?**

Little to none.

❑❑ **A primigravida is in labor for 15 hours, and her physical response to contractions is out of**

proportion to the intensity and duration of the contractions recorded on the external fetal monitor. How should you respond?

Check the accuracy of the fetal monitor by palpating the mother's abdomen while the contraction is occuring.

❑❑ **With the increase in new mothers being discharged less than 24 hours after delivery, what are some important teaching points you must address before the patient is released?**

Teaching regarding signs and symptoms of infection, retained placental fragments, uterine atony, and care of the infant.

❑❑ **What change in lochia would most likely be seen if placental fragments had been retained?**

An increase in the vaginal flow, a change in color to bright red, and an increase in clots.

❑❑ **A patient is progressing slowly in her labor, despite being dilated to 8 cm. You suddenly notice a bulge just above the symphysis. What does this indicate?**

The patient's bladder is full. She must either urinate or be catheterized.

❑❑ **What effect would emptying a patient's bladder have on the labor?**

It could speed up the fetal descent through the birth canal.

❑❑ **Prior to a cesarean section, why are patients often given glycopyrrolate (Robinul)?**

It is a parasympatholytic, which will decrease GI secretions.

❑❑ **What is the best way to prevent cold stress in a newborn that is having difficulty maintaining body temperature?**

A radiant heat warmer.

❑❑ **What is the most common reason why adolescent girls do not tell their parents about their unplanned pregnancy?**

Fear of rejection by the parents.

❑❑ **Why is it important to monitor the patient's urine output for amount and color when she is receiving an IV of magnesium sulfate?**

A decrease in urine output, or pink-tinged urine, can indicate potential renal damage.

❑❑ **What is ballottement?**

The manipulation of the fetal head by applying external pressure to the uterus.

❑❑ **If no ballottement is felt during the 4th to 5th months of pregnancy, what could this indicate?**

Oligohydramnios.

❑❑ **A patient undergoing a pitocin induction has contractions that are 1 1/2 minutes in length, occur every 90-100 seconds, with a fetal heart rate at 110 beats/minute. Should the induction continue?**

No. The fetus is showing signs of fetal distress (heart rate is too low), and the contractions are too long and too close together.

❑❑ **What is the one finding that indicates that a patient is in true labor?**

The cervix is 100% effaced and is beginning to dilate.

❑❑ **Being narcissistic and having a fascination with children is common during which trimester?**

The second.

❑❑ **A patient attempting a vaginal birth after a previous c-section (VBAC) suddenly has a sharp pain in her lower abdomen and the fetal monitor records no contractions. What is the possible cause?**

Uterine rupture.

❑❑ **What is the antidote of choice for magnesium sulfate toxicity?**

Calcium gluconate.

❑❑ **When is terbutaline (Brethine) used for pregnancy?**

For the treatment of preterm labor.

❑❑ **What position should you put a patient in when there is a prolapsed cord?**

The knee-chest position.

❑❑ **Why is this the best position?**

It reduces pressure on the cord so that there is no interruption of blood flow to the fetus.

❑❑ **What must you assess before giving pain medication to a patient in labor?**

Stage of labor, and the latest maternal and fetal vitals signs.

❑❑ **What are some of the disadvantages of epidural anesthesia?**

The chance of delivery by c-section may increase, it takes 10-20 minutes to take effect, maternal hypotension may result, and fetal heart rate may not be as variable.

❑❑ **When you notice variable decelerations on a fetal monitor, what should be the first intervention?**

Change maternal position, and/or administer oxygen.

❑❑ **Why is a newborn given plain, sterile water for the first feeding?**

If the initial feeding is aspirated, sterile water is less irritating to the lungs.

❒❒ **What is a hemangioma?**

A benign vascular tumor that may be present on the newborn.

❒❒ **Why would you have a patient who is about to receive an epidural anesthesia empty her bladder before the procedure?**

An epidural will lessen the sensation to void, so voiding now may decrease the need for catheterization later.

❒❒ **Why are newborns unable to maintain a stable body temperature?**

They have an immature vasomotor center, and are unable to shiver to increase body heat.

❒❒ **What nursing diagnoses are appropriate for a patient who is undergoing a c-section?**

Impaired gas exchange related to general anesthesia, pain, and alteration in comfort due to incisional pain.

❒❒ **A newborn who is 8 hours old is hyperactive, has a persistent, shrill cry, is jittery, and is yawning and sneezing. What is wrong with this infant?**

It is a drug-dependent neonate.

❒❒ **What is the major complication of epidural anesthesia?**

Maternal hypotension.

❒❒ **What interventions can minimize the hypotensive effects of epidural anesthesia?**

Prior to the procedure, adequately hydrate the patient and have her lie on her left side.

❒❒ **How often should vitals signs be monitored after epidural administration?**

Every 1-2 minutes for the first 15 minutes after the block.

❒❒ **If a pregnant woman has a monillial infection at the time of a vaginal delivery, what is the infant at risk for developing?**

Thrush.

❒❒ **What complication occurs if a preterm infant is overexposed to high oxygen levels?**

Retrolental fibroplasia.

❒❒ **What is a puerperal infection?**

An infection of the genital tract.

❒❒ **What are some of the signs and symptoms of a puerperal infection, and how long after delivery does it occur?**

Early symptoms include chills, fever, and flu-like symptoms. It can occur up to one month after delivery.

❑❑ **Why should you assess a newborn's palate with your index finger before feeding?**

To check for palate deformity.

❑❑ **What are the components of the Apgar scoring system?**

Tone, color, irritability, respiration, and heart rate.

❑❑ **How many units of insulin are you giving per hour if 1000 cc of D_5NS has 20 units of insulin, the solution set delivers 10 drops per ml/hour, and the IVAC is set to run at 100 ml/hour?**

$$\frac{\text{X units}}{\text{100 ml/hour}} = \frac{\text{20 units}}{\text{1000 ml}}$$

$$X = \frac{\text{20 units x 100 ml}}{\text{1000 ml}}$$

X = 2 units

❑❑ **What 2 components comprise gestational age determination?**

External characteristics and neuromuscular development.

❑❑ **Lochia serosa occurs after how many postpartum days?**

3-4.

❑❑ **What makes up lochia alba?**

Leukocytes, serum, and mucus.

❑❑ **What behavior would you expect in a newborn during the first period of reactivity?**

Awake, active, with a strong sucking reflex. This period usually lasts 30 minutes

❑❑ **You assess a 5-hour-old infant and find a rounded abdomen, normal temperature, irregular respiratory pattern, and cyanotic hands and feet. The infant has not voided or passed any meconium. Is there a cause for concern?**

No, these are normal findings in a 5-hour-old infant.

❑❑ **Two days after a normal delivery, a patient begins to cry for no apparent reason. What is happening?**

This transitory depression is caused by the change in hormone levels after delivery, which usually occurs 2 days after birth, and subsides within a week.

❑❑ **A patient develops premature labor at 30 weeks gestation. You immediately instruct her to lie down. You start an IV and give a bolus of 500 cc of solution. What is the rationale for these actions?**

Having the patient lie down may decrease pressure on the cervix, thereby decreasing the intensity and frequency of contractions. Hydrating the patient will decrease the release of ADH and oxytocin from the pituitary gland, which also stops labor from progressing.

❑❑ **How should you monitor a patient who is receiving oxytocin (Pitocin) to induce labor?**

Monitor placental circulation and fetal status, especially during contractions.

❑❑ **Where would you expect the fundal height to be one hour after birth?**

Midway between the umbilicus and the symphysis pubis.

❑❑ **At what rate does the fundal height generally descend into the pelvis?**

One finger's-breadth per day.

❑❑ **What factors must you consider when teaching a patient about postpartum weight loss in relation to breast feeding?**

The caloric needs of a nursing mother must be considered. Dieting should be avoided, in order to maintain adequate milk supply.

❑❑ **When is it safe for a patient to resume sexual activity after vaginal delivery?**

When the episiotomy has healed and the lochia had stopped. Usually 4-6 weeks.

❑❑ **A patient on ritodrine (Yutopar) for preterm labor begins complaining of jitters and nervousness. What is your best response?**

Ritodrine (Yutopar) can cause tremors and jittery feelings. You should assess whether the feelings are from the medication or from the pre-term labor.

❑❑ **What exercise is commonly taught to pregnant women to prevent problems with urination in the future?**

Kegel exercises.

❑❑ **A patient is concerned about her stretch marks and asks when they will go away. What is your best response?**

Stretch marks will eventually fade to a silvery-white color, but it is highly unlikely that they will completely disappear.

❑❑ **What are you looking for when performing a non-stress test?**

Spontaneous fetal movement associated with an increase in heart rate. This is considered a reactive, non-stress test, which indicates fetal well being.

❑❑ **What is the most common cause of hemorrhage after delivery?**

Uterine atony.

❑❑ **Why would you instruct a patient to massage her lower abdomen after delivery?**

To maintain a firm uterus, which will aid in the "clamping down" of blood vessels in the uterus, thereby preventing any further bleeding.

❑❑ **What position is the fetus in if the fontanel is toward the anterior portion of the pelvis?**

Occiput posterior.

❑❑ **When the fetus is in this position, what should you expect during labor?**

Intense back labor pains. Usually the fetus rotates to occiput anterior during labor.

❑❑ **What can you do to facilitate fetal rotation from occiput posterior to occiput anterior?**

Have the mother get on all fours.

❑❑ **A patient visits a family planning clinic to discuss her desire to have children. What should you do before performing a physical exam?**

Obtain a medical and sexual history.

❑❑ **Why do natural methods of birth control generally have a higher failure rate?**

Because these methods are based on knowing when ovulation occurs. Since this is difficult to determine accurately, the chance of miscalculation is high.

❑❑ **What primary structure in the female anatomy is involved in sexual arousal and orgasm?**

The clitoris.

❑❑ **When do most women ovulate?**

Two weeks before the beginning of the next period.

❑❑ **How long should a diaphragm be left in the vagina after sexual intercourse?**

6-8 hours.

❑❑ **A patient states that she would like a diaphragm, but has not been able to locate one in the stores. What is your response?**

The diaphragm is given by prescription only requiring it to be individually fitted. She will need to schedule an appointment with her physician for a fitting.

❑❑ **Besides sexual arousal, what is the function of foreplay?**

Increasing vaginal secretions.

❑❑ **Surgical sterilization of the male involves cutting what anatomical structure?**

The ductus deferens.

❑❑ **How long does it generally take for the sperm to reach the ovum under ideal conditions?**

1-5 minutes after ejaculation.

❑❑ **T/F: Sexual intercourse during menstruation is harmful.**

False.

❑❑ **How do oral contraceptives prevent pregnancy?**

They suppress FSH (follicle stimulating hormone) and LH (leutinizing hormone) release from the pituitary gland, thereby blocking ovulation.

❑❑ **When should the patient take her temperature when using the basal body temperature method of contraception?**

Every morning upon awakening and prior to any activity to avoid the temperature being influenced by other factors.

❑❑ **How are sperm propelled in the female?**

The sperms tail enables it to move on its own.

❑❑ **What does in vitro fertilization involve?**

The removal of a mature ovum from the female, fertilization with sperm in a petri dish, and implantation of the embryo into the female.

❑❑ **What is Chadwick's sign?**

A bluish coloring of the vaginal mucosa that occurs as early as 6 weeks gestation.

❑❑ **Name some of the presumptive signs of pregnancy.**

Breast tenderness, urinary frequency, fatigue, amenorrhea, vomiting, and nausea.

❑❑ **What are some of the probable (objective) signs of pregnancy?**

Goodell's sign, Chadwick's sign, Hegar's sign, abdominal enlargement, positive pregnancy test, and braxton-hicks contractions.

❑❑ **What is Goodell's sign?**

A softening of the cervix which occurs in pregnancy.

❑❑ **What are some of the positive signs of pregnancy?**

Fetal heart tones, ultrasound identification, and detection of fetal movement.

❑❑ **If a patient has positive objective signs of pregnancy but is not pregnant, what could be the cause?**

A hydatidiform mole pregnancy.

❑❑ **Where does fertilization usually occur?**

In the fallopian tubes.

❑❑ **An embryo that implants itself in an area other than the uterus is called what?**

Ectopic.

❑❑ **The radioimmunoassay pregnancy test is accurate within how many days after conception?**

7.

❑❑ **A radioimmunoassay detects the presence of what hormone?**

Human chorionic gonadotropin (HCG).

❑❑ **What is Naegle's rule?**

A formula to estimate the due date. It is the first day of last menstrual period, minus 3 months, plus 7 days.

❑❑ **How much alcohol consumption is safe during pregnancy?**

There is no generally accepted rule as to how much alcohol is safe. Therefore, the patient should be instructed to avoid alcohol during pregnancy.

❑❑ **What is the generally accepted amount of weight that a woman should gain during pregnancy?**

25-35 pounds.

❑❑ **What is Couvade syndrome?**

When the expectant father experiences some of the same pregnancy symptoms as the mother.

❑❑ **What measures can help to relieve the early morning nausea of pregnancy?**

Eating dry carbohydrate foods, such as crackers or toast.

❑❑ **Which foods most often tend to exacerbate morning sickness?**

Foods with a high fat content.

❑❑ **What should you do if a patient expresses fear over having a pelvic examination?**

Ask the patient to describe her fears. Knowing what she is afraid of will help you formulate a plan of care to help her deal with her fears.

❑❑ **What foods will help the absorption of iron tablets?**

Meat, and foods with vitamin C.

❑❑ **Why would you instruct a patient to drink 32 ounces of water within one hour prior to having an ultrasound?**

A full bladder will help in visualization of the fetus.

❑❑ **How does ultrasound work?**

High-frequency sound waves bounce off structures in the body, creating an image on a video screen.

❑❑ **What types of foods are high in iron?**

Meats, green vegetables, and most seafood.

❑❑ **Would it be safe for a patient to take a long automobile trip while in her second trimester?**

Yes, as long as no complications exist. However, she should stop every few hours to walk and stimulate circulation to her extremities.

❑❑ **What are some good sources of protein for the pregnant patient.**

Meat, fish, eggs, poultry, beans, nuts, milk, cheese, and wheat germ.

❑❑ **When is the pregnant patient tested for alpha-fetal protein (AFP) serum levels?**

Between 18-20 weeks gestation.

❑❑ **What is the significance of an elevated alpha-feto-protein (AFP) level?**

It can be an indication of neural tube defects such as spina bifida, anencephaly, multiple gestations, fetal death, abdominal wall defects, teratomas, and fetal distress.

❑❑ **An adolescent patient does not keep up with her prenatal visits. Why are these visits so important?**

There is a higher incidence of complications associated with adolescent pregnancies, including low birth weight infants, preterm labor, iron deficiency anemia, and cephalopelvic disproportion.

❑❑ **A patient who is 14 weeks pregnant is concerned because she has not felt the baby move yet. Is this a valid concern?**

No, most women do not experience quickening until 17-20 weeks gestation.

❑❑ **What is the purpose of Leopold's Maneuvers?**

To determine the position of the fetus.

❑❑ **Does an elevated AFP level always indicate that something is wrong with the fetus?**

No. Further evaluation is needed to determine the significance of a high level.

❑❑ **What are some abnormalities associated with a low AFP level?**

Genetic defects such as trisomy 13, 18, and 21.

❑❑ **A patient complains of urinary frequency at 38 weeks gestation. If a urinary tract infection is ruled out, what is the most likely cause?**

Lightening.

❑❑ **What is lightening?**

When the fetus descends into the pelvis, usually around 1-2 weeks before delivery.

❑❑ **Which foods are high in folic acid?**

Green, leafy vegetables such as spinach, broccoli, brussel sprouts, and asparagus.

❑❑ **How can varicose veins be prevented?**

Nothing can truly prevent them, but support hose, elevation of the lower extremities, and avoiding constrictive clothing can help.

❑❑ **What patient teaching can help relieve leg cramps during pregnancy?**

Push up on the toes and down on the knees when a cramp occurs. Elevating the legs and keeping them warm may also help.

❑❑ **What patient teaching can help relieve heartburn during pregnancy?**

Eat smaller frequent meals, avoid fatty foods, do not eat right before going to bed and elevate the head of the bed slightly.

❑❑ **A pregnant patient asks if she may take an antacid to relieve heartburn. Is this safe?**

Not really. Antacids are generally discouraged because of their high sodium content. However, they are not completely contraindicated if used infrequently.

❑❑ **When can the baby's heartbeat be heard through doppler?**

At 10-12 weeks gestation.

❑❑ **What teaching should be done to help a patient prepare her breasts for breast feeding prior to birth?**

Tugging and rolling the nipples between the fingers will help distribute natural lubrication to the nipples and form a protective layer of skin around the nipples, thereby decreasing their sensitivity.

❑❑ **The umbilical cord contains how many veins and arteries?**

One vein and 2 arteries.

❒❒ **What is the chromosome combination present in a female?**

XX.

❒❒ **How early can the sex of the fetus be determined by ultrasound?**

At 16 weeks gestation.

❒❒ **What 2 arteries supply the uterus with blood?**

The uterine and ovarian arteries.

❒❒ **What is the normal rate of blood loss during a vaginal delivery?**

500 ml.

❒❒ **What should you suspect if a patient complains of increased vaginal discharge and itching?**

Vaginal yeast infection.

❒❒ **What home remedies can pregnant patients use to treat hemorrhoids?**

Ice packs, topical ointments, sitz baths, a high fiber diet, and adequate fluid intake.

❒❒ **What is the purpose of amniotic fluid?**

It helps dilate the cervix in labor, protects the fetus from injury, and provides an even temperature for the fetus.

❒❒ **What is the primary cause of pain during the first stage of labor?**

Dilation of the cervix, pressure on adjacent structures, hypoxia of the uterine muscles during contractions, and stretching of the lower uterine segment.

❒❒ **What 2 structures form the placenta during the early stages of pregnancy?**

The chorionic villi and the decidual basalis.

❒❒ **What is the average weight of a term placenta?**

400-600 grams.

❒❒ **What functions does the placenta serve during pregnancy?**

Respiration, elimination, and nutrition.

❒❒ **What 3 hormones are produced by the placenta during pregnancy?**

Human placental lactogen, human chorionic gonadotrophin, and progesterone.

❑❑ **Does the placental vein or placental artery carry oxygen from the mother to the fetus?**

The placental vein.

❑❑ **What is a nuchal cord?**

An umbilical cord that is wrapped around the fetus' neck.

❑❑ **What are the characteristics of an inevitable abortion?**

Dilated cervix, bright red vaginal bleeding, and cramping.

❑❑ **For what is pentazocine hydrochloride (Talwin) used?**

It is used for pain control.

❑❑ **When is human anti-D globulin (RhoGAM) used?**

When the mother is Rh negative and the father is Rh positive.

❑❑ **Why is RhoGAM given?**

To prevent the mother from developing anti-Rh antibodies that could affect future pregnancies.

❑❑ **What is the purpose of administering butorphanol tartrate (Stadol)?**

To reduce discomfort.

❑❑ **A patient with a threatened abortion is sent home. What should you instruct her to do with her perineal pads, and why?**

The patient should save all her perineal pads so they can be inspected for the amount of bleeding and any tissue or clots passed.

❑❑ **What are the risk factors for pregnancy induced hypertension (PIH)?**

Primigravidas, family history of PIH, multiple gestations, diabetes mellitus, Rh incompatibility, lower socioeconomic status, and hydatidiform mole. Adolescents are at a higher risk than their older counterparts.

❑❑ **A patient with mild PIH at 34 weeks gestation complains that she has had a non-stop headache for the past 2 days. What should be your response?**

This could indicate worsening PIH. The patient should come to the clinic immediately for evaluation.

❑❑ **T/F: Overcooking vegetables destroys their vitamin C content.**

True.

❑❑ **What is pica?**

The ingestion of non-food substances, such as clay or dirt.

❑❑ What should you screen for in a patient with symptoms of pica?

Anemia. This is often a cause of pica.

❑❑ What are some of the symptoms of severe PIH?

Oliguria (< 400ml/24hrs), proteinuria, systolic BP above 160, and a diastolic BP above 100.

❑❑ What are the generally accepted rules for diagnosing mild PIH?

30 mm Hg or greater in systolic pressure, and 15 mm Hg or greater in diastolic pressure. Swelling of the hands, feet, and face may also be present.

❑❑ Why should mineral oil not be used to relieve constipation during pregnancy?

It prevents the absorption of fat soluble vitamins from the GI tract.

❑❑ When assigning a room to a patient with PIH, what factors should you consider?

The room should be near enough to monitor the patient closely, but not noisy or brightly lit. A quiet, calming environment for the patient is desired.

❑❑ What complications to the fetus are associated with PIH?

Stillbirth, prematurity, and intrauterine growth retardation.

❑❑ In a patient with PIH, what should you instruct the patient with regards to her activity at home?

Bedrest in the left recumbent position for most of the day.

❑❑ What is a common symptom of an impending seizure in a patient with PIH?

Severe headache.

❑❑ What is the antihypertensive drug of choice for a pregnant client with chronic hypertension?

Aldomet (methyldopa).

❑❑ What is the cure for PIH?

Delivery of the fetus.

❑❑ What special precautions should be assigned when admitting a patient with PIH?

Seizure precautions.

❑❑ How should you monitor a patient for hypermagnesemia?

Frequent assessment for diminished deep tendon reflexes.

❑❑ **What is HELLP syndrome?**

Hemolysis, elevated liver enzymes, and low platelet count.

❑❑ **What is the significance of the HELLP syndrome?**

Clients with HELLP syndrome and PIH have a high morbidity and mortality rate for themselves and their fetus.

❑❑ **If a client begins to convulse, what should be your first priority?**

Prevent injury from occurring to the patient first by placing her in a safe position, then begin with the ABC's by assessing the patency of the airway.

❑❑ **Before administering magnesium sulfate, what should you assess?**

Maternal respirations. $MgSO_4$ is a CNS depressant and will decrease respirations. If the maternal respirations are below 12-14 breaths per minute, the physician should be notified before starting the infusion.

❑❑ **A client enters the ED with heavy third trimester vaginal bleeding. What should be your first actions?**

Assess maternal and fetal vital signs.

❑❑ **What is the purpose of ritodrine (Yutopar)?**

To stop preterm labor.

❑❑ **What is a contraindication to ritodrine (Yutopar)?**

Cervical dilation.

❑❑ **When assessing for abruptio placentae, for what should you look?**

A rigid board-like abdomen, with dark red painful vaginal bleeding.

❑❑ **What is the common cause of abruptio placentae?**

No common cause has been found.

❑❑ **The patient with suspected placenta previa suddenly develops severe vaginal bleeding. The initial nursing action should include:**

Notify the doctor, start an IV infusion to replace the lost fluid volume, then frequent monitoring of the maternal and fetal vital signs.

❑❑ **What is complete placenta previa?**

When the placenta completely covers the cervical os.

❒❒ **When monitoring fetal heart rate, what is the best position of the doppler on the maternal abdomen?**

Over the back of the fetus.

❒❒ **What is the normal fetal heart rate?**

120-160 beats per minute

❒❒ **What is a common side effect of ritodrine (Yutopar)?**

Tachycardia.

❒❒ **What other side effects can occur as a result of ritodrine (Yutopar) therapy?**

Occasional PVCs, increased BP, palpitations, tremors, nausea and vomiting, and shortness of breath.

❒❒ **A patient asks why she needs an ultrasound prior to having an amniocentesis. What is the reasoning behind this?**

An ultrasound is used to locate the placenta, position of the fetus, and any pockets of amniotic fluid prior to performing the amniocentesis to determine the best location to insert the needle.

❒❒ **What should you look for when assessing for placenta previa?**

Painless bright red vaginal bleeding.

❒❒ **What does a "negative contraction" result indicate in a stress test?**

A normal result. No fetal heart rate decelerations were detected during a contraction.

❒❒ **What does a "positive contraction" result indicate in a stress test?**

An indication of fetal compromise. Fetal decelerations are detected in response to stress (contractions). This result could cause the physician to choose a c-section delivery in order to avoid undue stress to the fetus from a vaginal delivery.

❒❒ **After the amniocentesis, what symptom should you instruct the patient to report immediately?**

Vaginal bleeding.

❒❒ **T/F: An insulin dependent diabetic should be aware that her insulin needs will most likely decrease as the pregnancy progresses.**

False. Insulin needs may be 4 times as high due to the presence of human placental lactogen, estrogen, and progesterone, which are insulin antagonists.

❒❒ **During the postpartum period, how will the insulin needs change for a pregnant diabetic?**

They will fall significantly.

❑❑ **Where should the nurse place the tokodynamometer for the best results?**

At the top of the fundus.

❑❑ **How does the tokodynamometer work?**

It records the intensity of contractions by sensing the rise in the abdomen when the uterus contracts. The pressure of the abdominal contraction presses against the transducer recording the intensity of the contraction.

❑❑ **What does a non-reactive non-stress test result mean?**

The fetus had less than 2 heart rate accelerations associated with movement during a 10 to 20 minute period. This result could indicate fetal compromise.

❑❑ **What is the purpose of a contraction stress test?**

To determine fetal compromise during contractions.

❑❑ **A client in her second trimester complains of frequent vomiting to the point where she cannot keep anything down. You tell her to try eating crackers and call back tomorrow. Is this good advice?**

No. Vomiting in the second trimester, especially when it is excessive, needs immediate follow-up to rule out any complications. You should always ask detailed questions about the vomiting such as how often, last time food or fluids stayed down, and urine output.

❑❑ **What procedures can be used to diagnose an ectopic pregnancy?**

Culdocentesis, ultrasound, laparoscopy, or laparotomy.

❑❑ **What is a culdocentesis and how can it diagnose an ectopic pregnancy?**

If bleeding occurs into the pelvic cavity as a result of the ectopic, then aspiration of non-clotting blood in the cul-de-sac of Douglas (culdocentesis) will confirm the diagnosis.

❑❑ **T/F: A fetal biophysical profile is a long and extensive test that takes several weeks before results can be calculated.**

False. This test is easy, non-invasive, and results can be obtained immediately once all the data is collected.

❑❑ **What is one of the first symptoms of hypoglycemia?**

Nervousness.

❑❑ **What are some of the complications of pregnant diabetics?**

Infection, polyhydramnios, ketoacidosis, large birth weight infants, and congenital abnormalities.

❑❑ **While in labor, how often should the diabetic client have her blood glucose checked?**

Hourly.

❑❑ **When a client has hyperemesis gravidarum, what electrolyte may be depleted?**

Potassium.

❑❑ **What is the most common cause of an ectopic pregnancy?**
Past history of pelvic inflammatory disease.

❑❑ **What is the primary cause of premature rupture of membranes?**

There is no primary identifiable cause, but it has been associated with infection, multiple gestations, trauma, and an incompetent cervix.

❑❑ **What symptoms would lead the nurse to suspect a molar pregnancy?**

Absence of fetal heart rate, brownish vaginal discharge, uterine enlargement that is greater that the estimated gestational age, elevated HCG levels, PIH, and the passage of hydropic vessels.

❑❑ **A patient with hyperemesis gravidarum should be assessed for what potential complication?**

Dehydration.

❑❑ **What symptoms would the nurse expect if a tubal rupture were to occur from an ectopic pregnancy?**

A sharp, severe, knife-like pain in the lower quadrant, often associated with referred shoulder pain.

❑❑ **What is the most accurate method for home glucose monitoring?**

Accucheck machine. Urine glucose testing is not as reliable.

❑❑ **A client who has been exercising regularly before she became pregnant wishes to continue her exercising during the pregnancy. Is this safe?**

Yes, as long as the patient does not over-exert herself. There should be no harm to the fetus if the patient continues to exercise at the level she was at before pregnancy.

❑❑ **Following a dilation and curettage (D&C), you should assess for what potential complication?**

Hemorrhage.

❑❑ **Following the evacuation of a hydatidiform mole, the patient should to be monitored for what type of complication over the next 1-2 years?**

The development of a choriocarcinoma.

❑❑ **Following the evacuation of a molar pregnancy, the patient asks when she will be able to get pregnant again. What is your response?**

The patient should not get pregnant for 1-2 years while her HCG levels are monitored for the possible development of choriocarcinoma.

❑❑ **You should be aware of what common emotion felt by the mother after the delivery of a premature infant?**

Guilt. The mother often feels she did something wrong to cause the premature delivery.

❑❑ **A client is admitted at 35 weeks gestation with premature rupture of membranes. The physician orders the administration of betamethasone. Why?**

Betamethasone will accelerate the development of fetal lungs.

❑❑ **What are some of the possible side effects of betamethasone therapy?**

Weight gain, increased risk of infection, GI bleeding, initiation of lactation, edema, and hypoglycemia in the neonate.

❑❑ **A patient is admitted with hyperemesis gravidarum. You do a urine dipstick to assess for what substance?**

Acetone.

❑❑ **A client in active labor at 39 weeks gestation is admitted, and you perform Leopold's Maneuver. Why?**

To identify fetal presentation and position.

❑❑ **What is "active relaxation" during labor?**

Relaxing the uninvolved muscles during labor while contracting a specific group of muscles and using deep breathing techniques to help ease the pain of labor.

❑❑ **When a patient uses personalized concentration points or ideas during labor, what purpose does this serve?**

It is a method of distraction used to ease the pain of labor.

❑❑ **What is the average length of labor for a primigravida?**

12-14 hours.

❑❑ **A patient expresses the urge to push, but her cervix is not fully dilated. What should you do?**

Do not allow her to push and instruct her in the "pant-pant" method of breathing during a contraction.

❑❑ **If a patient was allowed to push when the cervix was not fully dilated, what could happen?**

Increased swelling to the cervix which could make labor more difficult while also causing bruising and swelling to the presenting part of the infant.

❑❑ **What happens during the transition phase of labor?**

Contractions increase in frequency, intensity, and duration.

❑❑ **What test can you perform to determine if the membranes have ruptured?**

A nitrazine test on vaginal fluid.

❑❑ **What is the nitrazine test?**

A test using nitrazine paper to determine the pH of the vaginal fluid. A pH above 6.5 indicates the membranes have ruptured, while a pH below 6.0 represents normal vaginal fluid.

❑❑ **What color will the nitrazine paper turn if the test is positive for amniotic fluid?**

Blue.

❑❑ **While a patient is holding her infant after birth she begins to cry. You would interpret this reaction in what way?**

A normal response to the emotional process of childbirth.

❑❑ **An Apgar score between 4 and 6 indicates what condition?**

Fair.

❑❑ **What is the highest Apgar score an infant can receive?**

10.

❑❑ **What 2 time intervals after birth is the Apgar score assessed in the neonate?**

1 and 5 minutes after birth.

❑❑ **During the transition stage of labor, what is the most important thing you can provide for the patient?**

Emotional support and encouragement.

❑❑ **What is the most reliable sign that the placenta is about to be delivered?**

Lengthening of the cord outside of the vagina indicating detachment of the placenta from the uterine wall.

❑❑ **Why is oxytocin (Pitocin) given after delivery of the placenta?**

It promotes uterine contractions and helps to control postpartum bleeding.

❑❑ **How soon can breast feeding be started after delivery?**

Immediately.

❑❑ **Why is there no concern for first testing the patency of the esophagus before breast feeding?**

Unlike formula, Colostrum is not irritating to the lungs if aspirated, so there is no danger if the esophagus is not patent.

❒❒ **What anatomical landmarks are used to determine the descent of the fetal presenting part?**

The ischial spines.

❒❒ **If the presenting part is said to be at +1, what does this mean?**

The presenting part is 1 cm below the ischial spines.

❒❒ **What symptoms would indicate to the nurse that the patient is hyperventilating during labor?**

A complaint of feeling dizzy, short of breath, elevated blood pressure, tingling of the hands and feet, and feeling lightheaded.

❒❒ **What is effleurage?**

Light stroking of the skin often used in Lamaze to promote relaxation.

❒❒ **Is the patient allowed to walk while in labor?**

If no complications exist, the patient may walk during the first stage of labor.

❒❒ **T/F: When a patient hyperventilates you will most likely see symptoms of respiratory acidosis.**

False. Respiratory alkalosis occurs due to the depletion of carbon dioxide.

❒❒ **What is a low forceps delivery?**

When the fetal presenting part is at +2 station or higher.

❒❒ **What is a midforceps delivery?**

When the fetal presenting part is engaged but above +2 station.

❒❒ **At what level is forceps delivery not indicated?**

If the fetal skull is at the level of the ischial spines.

❒❒ **What should you assess after the membranes rupture and the neonate is at +1 station?**

Assess the color, odor, and consistency of the amniotic fluid.

❒❒ **If the head were not engaged and the membranes rupture, what would be your first priority?**

Check for prolapse of the cord.

❒❒ **What is the normal color of amniotic fluid?**

Straw colored.

❑❑ **If the amniotic fluid is greenish or brown colored, what could this indicate?**

The color of the fluid could indicate the presence of meconium due to the fetus suffering a hypoxic event.

❑❑ **T/F: Following the administration of an epidural block, your first priority is to assess the patient's level of anesthesia.**

False. Although this is important, the priority is to assess the blood pressure which can fall after administration of an epidural.

❑❑ **A husband becomes frustrated when a patient reaches the transition stage and begins to lose control. What advice should the nurse give?**

Keep supporting the patient. Her reaction is normal and she needs help in focusing on the labor and maintaining control.

❑❑ **At the onset of labor, you notice a small amount of bloody vaginal discharge (show). What action should you take?**

A bloody show usually indicates cervical dilation; therefore you should do a vaginal exam.

❑❑ **What is the basic premise of the Gate Control pain theory?**

Pain can be blocked at the spinal cord by halting the impulses before they reach the brain, thus pain is not perceived.

❑❑ **During the active phase of labor, how often should maternal blood pressure be monitored?**

Every hour between contractions unless there are signs of hypo or hypertension.

❑❑ **What type of decelerations are associated with cord compression?**

Variable decelerations.

❑❑ **If early decelerations are seen early in labor and they mirror the contractions, what could be the cause?**

Cephalopelvic disproportion.

❑❑ **A patient shows signs of hyperventilation during labor. What should you do?**

Instruct the patient to slow her breathing and if necessary, have her breathe into a paper bag.

❑❑ **Before starting a patient on IV oxytocin (Pitocin) for labor induction, what should you do in regards to assessing the fetus?**

Check the baseline heart rate which will give an indication of fetal distress once contractions start.

❑❑ **After the membranes have ruptured, you note frequent variable decelerations. What should you do?**

Continue monitoring and see if a change in position will help. Variable decelerations are common after the membranes have ruptured due to cord compression.

❒❒ **To improve cardiac emptying and oxygenation during labor, what simple measures can you implement?**

Have the patient lie on her left side and administer oxygen.

❒❒ **What is the cause of late decelerations?**

Inadequate placental perfusion.

❒❒ **A patient's water breaks and it is meconium stained. What would this indicate to you?**

The fetus has suffered a hypoxic event. Close monitoring of fetal well being is indicated.

❒❒ **When a client receives a pudendal block, where will most of the pain relief be concentrated?**

In the perineum.

❒❒ **If the amniotic fluid shows evidence of meconium staining, what will the physician most likely do immediately after delivery?**

Suction the oropharynx immediately after the head is delivered and before the chest is delivered.

❒❒ **What is the rational for suctioning the infant before the chest is delivered?**

If the chest is compressed in the vagina, the infant will not inhale. Once delivered, the infant will inhale and the potential for meconium aspiration is greater.

❒❒ **You determine a postpartum client has uterine atony. What problem does this lead to?**

Postpartum hemorrhage.

❒❒ **What essential data is collected when admitting a client to the labor unit?**

Frequency, intensity, and duration of contractions, when labor began, are the membranes ruptured, due date, primigravida or multigravida, last meal, allergies, prenatal care, and vital signs.

❒❒ **Why is it of significance to know if the patient is a multigravida or primigravida?**

It could indicate the duration of labor and the patient's response to the labor process.

❒❒ **A patient in labor states she can feel the baby coming. What is your first action?**

Inspect the perineum and assess for crowning.

❒❒ **What are the complications related to deep suctioning of the neonate?**

Stimulation of the vagus nerve, damage to mucous membranes, and hypoxia.

❑❑ **If the vagus nerve is stimulated during suctioning, what would you expect to see?**

A drop in heart rate.

❑❑ **Approximately 15 minutes after a normal delivery, the patient complains of feeling chilled and begins to shiver. What should you do?**

Provide warm blankets. This is a common reaction after delivery.

❑❑ **If insulin is required during labor, what is the preferred method of administration?**

Intravenous.

❑❑ **The fetus is at -2 station and the membranes rupture. For what is the patient at risk?**

Prolapsed cord.

❑❑ **How do you determine if a prolapsed cord exists?**

Perform a vaginal exam.

❑❑ **A client who received lumbar epidural anesthesia cannot detect when a contraction occurs. How will she patient know when to push?**

You or the coach will palpate the fundus, inform the patient when a contraction is occurring, and instruct her to push.

❑❑ **When should an oxytocin (Pitocin) infusion be discontinued?**

At signs of fetal distress, contractions longer that 60 seconds, or less than 2 minutes apart.

❑❑ **What are the advantages of an episiotomy?**

It facilitates the delivery of the fetus, it prevents tearing of the perineum, and it prevents undo stretching of the perineal muscles.

❑❑ **What does the term "dizygotic twins" mean?**

Fertilization occurred with 2 separate ova and sperm. This is also known as fraternal twins.

❑❑ **The delivery of a full term neonate is imminent and there is no physician available. What should you do?**

Prepare to deliver the neonate on your own.

❑❑ **When delivering the neonate, should you deliver the head between contractions or during a contraction?**

Between contractions. This will prevent the head from being delivered too suddenly, thus preventing a possible tearing of the perineum.

❑❑ **Once the head is delivered, what should you check for?**

Check for cord position. If it is around the neck it should be pulled gently and slipped over the head.

❑❑ **Once you have checked for the cord, how should the rest of the body be delivered?**

Apply gentle traction on the anterior shoulder, advising the patient not to push.

❑❑ **How do you know when to deliver the placenta?**

Watch for cord lengthening, a slight gush of darkened blood, or a change in fundal shape.

❑❑ **What could happen if the cord is pulled on before the placenta has separated?**

Uterus inversion, or retained placental fragments.

❑❑ **What are the complications that you should watch for in the post-mature infant after delivery?**

Hypoglycemia, meconium aspiration, polycythemia, and cold stress.

❑❑ **What are the complications of a pudendal block that can be seen in the neonate?**

Bradycardia, hypotonia, decreased responsiveness, and seizures due to high levels of anesthetic in the infant's blood stream.

❑❑ **What is thought to be the cause of complications seen in the neonate after a pudendal block?**

Accidental injection of the fetal scalp.

❑❑ **A patient asks why she needs to have a Foley catheter inserted before her c-section. What is the reasoning for this?**

To keep the bladder empty at all times during surgery, reducing the risk of bladder injury, and to aid in elimination which is affected by spinal/epidural anesthesia.

❑❑ **What is the purpose of nalbuphine (Nubain) when given during labor?**

It is an analgesic used for pain relief.

❑❑ **How can a patient avoid performing the valsalva maneuver while pushing?**

Exhale slowly while pushing rather than holding her breath.

❑❑ **What should be suspected if a patient has been in active labor for 2 hours with no change in dilation or effacement?**

Cephalopelvic disproportion.

❑❑ **What is the measurement used to determine if the size of a patient's pelvis is adequate for vaginal delivery?**

The true conjugate or obstetric conjugate measurement.

❒❒ **Is it safe for a patient who has herpes simples type 2 to deliver vaginally?**

Yes, if there are no lesions present. If lesions are present, a cesarean section should be performed.

❒❒ **What effect can analgesia have on the monitor readings of the fetus during labor?**

Minimal variability but the baseline heart rate should remain within normal limits.

❒❒ **What should you assess a patient for after a cesarean delivery?**

Uterine atony. This is more common after a c-section than after a vaginal delivery.

❒❒ **What is a patient who has a precipitous labor at risk for as a result of the labor process?**

Laceration of the soft tissues, uterine rupture, and excessive uterine bleeding.

❒❒ **When obtaining a signature for an elective c-section, a husband signs the form for his wife because he is the biological father of the child. Is this valid?**

No. As with any surgery, only the patient can give informed consent. If the patient is unable to sign, then it would be permitted for the husband to sign in the case of an emergency.

❒❒ **What is polyhydramnios?**

Excessive amniotic fluid.

❒❒ **What could be a possible cause of bright yellow amniotic fluid?**

Rh sensitization. The yellow color is the result of fetal anemia and bilirubin.

❒❒ **What is an amniotic fluid embolism?**

When amniotic fluid leaks into the maternal bloodstream.

❒❒ **What are the causes of an amniotic fluid embolism?**

Difficult labor, or hyperstimulation of the uterus.

❒❒ **What are the symptoms of an amniotic fluid embolism?**

Respiratory distress, acute hemorrhage, circulatory collapse, tachycardia, hypotension, cyanosis, and chest pain.

❒❒ **What should be your first action when uterine cord prolapse occurs?**

Relieve pressure on the cord by changing the patient's position.

❒❒ **What is the best technique for preventing breast engorgement when breast feeding?**

Frequent, regular, emptying of the breasts.

❑❑ **A patient is diagnosed with infectious mastitis. Can she continue breast feeding?**

Yes, breastfeeding is encouraged to help prevent breast engorgement. There is no danger of passing the infection to the infant.

❑❑ **For RhoGAM to be effective, when should it be administered in the postpartum period?**

Within 72 hours after delivery.

❑❑ **According to the American Academy of Pediatrics, how long should an infant be on breast milk or formula?**

Until one year of age.

❑❑ **Why is cow's milk not recommended for infants as their only means of nutrition under one year of age?**

Cow's milk is poorly digested due to its high protein content. After 6 months of age, an infant may have cow's milk as long as it does not account for more than 65% of their caloric intake.

❑❑ **What does the "taking in" phase consist of during the postpartum period?**

It usually lasts 3 days, and the patient is concerned with meeting her own needs rather than controlling everything in her environment.

❑❑ **What is the final phase of the postpartum psychological adaptation?**

Letting go.

❑❑ **How often should a patient breast feed her baby after delivery?**

Every 2-3 hours is recommended until her milk supply is established.

❑❑ **A patient is concerned when she changes her infants' diaper soon after delivery and finds a small amount of blood tinged drainage from the baby's vagina. Should she be concerned?**

No. This is common in newborn girls and is thought to be caused from the mother's estrogen influence while in utero.

❑❑ **Why is Erythromycin ointment placed in the neonates eyes soon after birth?**

Prophylactic treatment against Neisseria gonorrhea and chlamydia trachomatis.

❑❑ **What is the correct procedure for placing eye ointment in the neonates eyes?**

Instill into the lower conjunctival sac starting at the inner canthus.

❑❑ **Soon after delivery, the patient asks to go to the bathroom. Is this accepted?**

As long as the patient had a local anesthetic and the nurse assists, there should be no reason why the patient cannot use the bathroom.

❑❑ With the bottle fed infant, how much formula should you instruct the patient to prepare ahead of time?

No more than 24 hours worth.

❑❑ What is the usual treatment for infectious mastitis?

Heating pad to the breast, antibiotics, analgesics, and increased fluid intake.

❑❑ What is best position to place a patient in to assess the episiotomy?

The Sim's position.

❑❑ How many calories per ounce does human milk and formula contain?

20 calories per ounce.

❑❑ Does breast size determine the patient's ability to nurse effectively?

No. Hormones such as prolactin and sufficient glandular tissue in the breast plays the biggest role in breast feeding.

❑❑ What other factors can affect the amount of milk produced when breast feeding?

Emptying of the breasts, suckling, diet, rest, exercise, stress, and level of contentment with the breast feeding process.

❑❑ When assessing a patient after delivery, you observe ecchymosis and swelling in and around the perineum. What measures can relieve some of this pain and swelling?

Ice bag to the perineum for the first 24 hours, sitz baths, and administration of analgesics.

❑❑ What is the muscle of choice for intramuscular injections in the neonate?

The vastus lateralis.

❑❑ Why is phytonadione (AquaMephyton) given to the neonate after delivery?

To assist in clotting.

❑❑ What hormone is responsible for the let-down reflex in breast feeding?

Oxytocin.

❑❑ What hormone is responsible for milk production?

Prolactin.

❑❑ **What is the TPAL method of pregnancy documentation?**

T: Number of term infants,
P: Number of preterm infants,
A: Number of abortions,
L: Number of currently living children.

❑❑ **A postpartum client is placed on heparin therapy for treatment of thrombophlebitis. What medication should you have on hand to counteract the effects of heparin if needed?**

Protamine sulfate.

❑❑ **A neonate suddenly extends his arms with hands open and then moves them into an embracing position when startled. Is this normal?**

Yes. this is the Moro, or startle reflex that disappears at about 3 months of age.

❑❑ **What is the approximate distance a newborn can see?**

About 9-12 inches.

❑❑ **What precautions should you take when a postpartum client starts ambulating?**

Fall precautions and close monitoring should be done due to the risk of syncopy, especially the first few times out of bed.

❑❑ **When assessing a patient's readiness to breast feed and her chances of successful feeding, what is the most important factor you should look for?**

The patient's motivation and attitude towards breast feeding.

❑❑ **T/F: Breast fed neonates do not swallow as much air as bottle fed neonates and therefore do not need to be burped.**

False. Even though breast fed infants swallow less air than bottle fed infants, they still need to be burped.

❑❑ **When attempting to catheterize a patient, you feel some resistance. What should you do?**

Ask the patient to bear down as if urinating. The catheter could have caused a bladder spasm and bearing down may relieve this.

❑❑ **What is the lochia called that occurs for 2-3 days after delivery?**

Lochia rubra.

❑❑ **How long should a client wait to become pregnant after receiving a rubella vaccine?**

3 months.

❑❑ **What is the Betke-Kleihauer test?**

A test that determines if a greater than usual fetal - maternal blood mix occurred. It is used in Rh incompatibility cases to determine if another dose of RhoGAM is needed.

❒❒ **What space is the needle injected into with spinal anesthesia?**

The subarachnoid space.

❒❒ **What are the side effects of spinal anesthesia?**

Spinal headache, hypotension, total spinal blockade involving even respiratory paralysis, and bladder dysfunction.

❒❒ **An adolescent new mother has special emotional needs during the postpartum period. How can you assist in meeting these needs?**

Offer praise and encouragement for her mothering skills. Instructions should be simple and straightforward. Boosting self-confidence and self-esteem are important.

❒❒ **Two weeks after birth, a patient is worried because her infant is demanding to feed more often than his usual 4-hour schedule. What should you say?**

A normal growing infant who suddenly demands more feedings is more than likely going through a growth spurt. Increase the feedings to meet this demand.

❒❒ **Why do infants spit up their formula/breast milk after feeding?**

There are several thoughts on this. The most accepted reasons are that infants have an immature cardiac sphincter, or that the feeding is regurgitated when a gas bubble is released. Initially it was believed to be due to excessive mucous and gastric irritation from substances in the stomach at birth.

❒❒ **Can a nursing mother stop producing breast milk when she decides to stop breast feeding?**

Gradual weaning by eliminating one feeding at a time will eventually slow milk production until feedings are eventually eliminated.

❒❒ **What is the best method of caring for an infant's umbilical cord?**

Clean with rubbing alcohol. This promotes drying and helps decrease the risk of infection.

❒❒ **After delivery, should a mother see the infant that she has placed for adoption?**

It should be left up to the patient whether she wants to see the infant or not. It often assists in the grief process if she can hold the infant and participate in some of his care before releasing him to the adoptive parents.

❒❒ **Two days after her c-section, the patient complains of gas pains. What are some ways to help relieve these pains?**

Increase activity, avoid very hot, cold, or carbonated beverages, and if necessary, medications may be used to relieve gas.

❑❑ **Why is talking to an infant important even though they cannot understand you?**

It provides sensory stimulation, assists in language development, and promotes bonding between parent and child.

❑❑ **Following delivery, the patient is having difficulty voiding. What causes this?**

Edema in the area of the lower urinary tract from the trauma of labor and delivery.

❑❑ **Why should you assess for bladder distention closely following delivery?**

The edema in the lower urinary tract often decreases the sensation to void leading to bladder distention and insufficient bladder emptying.

❑❑ **What can be done to prevent nipple soreness?**

Air dry nipples after feeding, expose them to light, place as much of the areola as possible into the infant's mouth, change positions when breast feeding so the same area of the nipple is not used each time, feed on demand so the infant is not so hungry that his suck is too strong.

❑❑ **What teaching should you do with a patient in regards to taking medications while breastfeeding?**

Avoid all non-prescription medication until talking with your doctor. Always inform the physician that you are breastfeeding if medication is prescribed.

❑❑ **A patient is worried she will "spoil" her baby by holding him too much. How should you respond?**

Contrary to many beliefs, newborns can never be held too much. They respond to tactile stimulation and this helps them develop trust in their caregiver.

❑❑ **Why do women experience cramps when they are breastfeeding?**

Oxytocin is released during breastfeeding causing uterine cramps. This process helps the uterus return to its normal size and prevents uterine atony.

❑❑ **A patient is prescribed medication approved for use during breastfeeding. When should she take the medication in relation to feeding time?**

Right after breastfeeding. Drug concentrations are highest soon after they are taken.

❑❑ **A patient delivers a stillborn and asks to see her infant. Why has this been found to be helpful?**

It assists in beginning the grieving process. Taking a picture of the infant, if the mother desires, may also be helpful.

❑❑ **What is the best type of visual stimulation for a neonate?**

The human face. Infants like to look at the eyes which provide a dark object against a lighter background.

❑❑ **What is the best method for manual expression of milk?**

Using your thumb and forefinger, compress and release the breast at the edge of the areola, being careful not to irritate the areola by rubbing it.

❒❒ **After feeding, what is the best position to place a neonate?**

On the right side to aid in digestion.

❒❒ **If you find a patient's fundus to be "boggy", what should you do before calling the M.D.?**

Massage the fundus.

❒❒ **The first time out of bed a patient experiences a gush of lochia rubra. Should you be concerned?**

No. Pooling of lochia is normal and discharge is expected to increase, especially the first time out of bed. However, if the bleeding is severe and bright red, notify the M.D.

❒❒ **Following a c-section, you decide to advance the patient's diet from NPO to clear liquids based on what finding?**

The presence of bowel sounds.

❒❒ **Besides taking her antibiotics until gone, what other teaching should you do with a patient in regards to the treatment of cystitis?**

Drink lots of fluids, wear cotton underwear, and void frequently.

❒❒ **What genetic abnormality is the cause of Down's Syndrome?**

An extra chromosome in the 21st pair.

❒❒ **Before administering methylergonovine maleate (Methergine), what should you check?**

Blood pressure. Methergine can cause hypertension.

❒❒ **How can you distinguish vomiting from regurgitation in the neonate?**

Vomited material has a curdled appearance and a sour odor. Regurgitated material has almost no odor and occurs immediately after feeding.

❒❒ **What feelings characterize the "taking hold" phase of the postpartum period?**

Fear and concern over her ability to care for her child.

❒❒ **What is the fluid that begins to drain from the nipples during the last trimester of pregnancy and initially after delivery?**

Colostrum.

❒❒ **What 2 factors in the lactating mothers diet are important in order to keep milk production up?**

Calories and fluids.

❑❑ **What action by the mother stimulates the neonate to open his mouth to nurse?**

Lightly brushing the nipple across his mouth.

❑❑ **Why is breast milk not to be stored in glass containers?**

The immunoglobulins stick to glass.

❑❑ **How long can breast milk be stored?**

In the freezer for 2 months, and in the refrigerator for 48 hours.

❑❑ **How many calories per day, per pound of body weight does the neonate need to consume?**

50 to 55 calories per pound, per day (117 calories per Kg of weight per day).

❑❑ **What is the most likely contributing factor to puerperal infections?**

Multiple vaginal exams and vaginal trauma from labor and delivery.

❑❑ **One week after delivery, a patient complains of frequent crying for no apparent reason and feelings of depression. This is most likely the result of what?**

Postpartum depression caused by the rapid change in hormone levels.

❑❑ **Describe how true labor differs from false labor.**

True labor produces regular rhythmic contractions, abdominal discomfort. Leaveout progressive fetal dissent, bloody show, and progressive cervical effacement and dilatation.

❑❑ **When should self-exam of the breast be performed?**

It should be performed on the 5th and 7th day after the first day of the menstrual period when hormonal affects, which can cause breast lumps and tenderness, are reduced.

❑❑ **In a post-menopausal woman recieving cyclical estrogen, what is the best time to perform a breast self- examination?**

The last day that she is not taking the estrogen.

❑❑ **What are the tocolytic agents used to treat pre-term labor?**

Terbutaline sulfate (Brethine), ritodrine hydrochloride (Yutopar) and magnesium sulfate.

❑❑ **What is the recommended weight gain during pregnancy?**

25-35 pounds.

❑❑ **What are indications that the mother's milk supply is adequate for a breast-fed infant?**

The child will appear content, have good skin turgor, an adequate number of wet diapers, and normal weight gain.

❒❒ T/F: A nurse should wear gloves when handling a neonate until the first bath is given.

True. The infant will be contaminated with body fluids so universal precautions should be used.

❒❒ Strawberry hemangiomas are raised red birth marks that may continue to spread up to age one. Complete shrinkage and absorption may take up to how long?

7-10 years.

❒❒ What is caput succedaneum?

Scalp edema that develops during labor and delivery which resolves spontaneously and presents no danger to the neonate.

❒❒ To establish a milk supply pattern, how often should a mother breast feed her infant?

Every 4 hours during the first month, or 8-12 times a day (demand feeding).

❒❒ Upon delivery, how is heat loss prevented in the neonate?

By placing the neonate under a radiant warmer during suctioning, and initial assessment.

❒❒ What blood vessels are contained in the umbilical cord?

Two arteries and one vein.

❒❒ What is the average weight of a neonate?

5-9 pounds.

❒❒ What is the average length of a neonate?

18-22 inches.

❒❒ What is the average head circumference of a neonate?

13-14 inches.

❒❒ What is the normal temperature range for a neonate?

98-99 degrees Fahrenheit.

❒❒ What is the average apical pulse of a neonate?

120-160 beats per minute.

❒❒ What is the normal respiratory rate of a neonate?

40-60 breaths per minute.

❑❑ **When does the anterior fontanel close?**

12-18 months of age.

❑❑ **When does the posterior fontanel usually close?**

2 months of age.

❑❑ **What is a positive Babinski reflex?**

Toe fanning when the sole is stroked from heel to toe.

❑❑ **A Babinski reflex is present in a neonate up to what age?**

18 months.

❑❑ **How do you assess the rooting reflex?**

You touch a finger to the neonate's cheek or corner of its mouth. Normally, the neonate turns its head towards the stimulus, opens their mouth, and searches for the stimulus.

❑❑ **What is Goodell's sign?**

Softening of the cervix during pregnancy.

❑❑ **What is a safe level of alcohol intake for pregnant women?**

None.

❑❑ **What is the most ideal pelvis shape for delivery?**

A gynecoid pelvis.

❑❑ **When do heroin withdrawal symptoms occur in a neonate?**

Several hours to 4 days after birth.

❑❑ **When do methadone withdrawal symptoms occur in a neonate?**

7 days to several weeks after birth.

❑❑ **What is the first sign of toxic shock syndrome?**

Rapid onset of a high fever.

❑❑ **At 20-weeks gestation, where should the fundus of the uterus be?**

At the umbilicus.

❑❑ **What is the definition of a threatened abortion?**

When vaginal bleeding is present without cervical dilation.

❑❑ **What is the definition of a premature infant?**

An infant born before the end of the 37th week of gestation.

❑❑ **To what does the term "gravida" refer?**

The number of pregnancies, regardless of their outcome.

❑❑ **To what does the term "para" refer?**

The number of viable young.

❑❑ **What is an ectopic pregnancy?**

A pregnancy that implants outside of the uterus.

❑❑ **What is Cullen's sign?**

A bluish-discoloration around the umbilicus.

❑❑ **What does Cullen's sign indicate?**

Intra-abdominal or peritoneal bleeding.

❑❑ **What is the definition of a low-birth-weight infant?**

1,500-2,500 grams (3 pounds, 5 ounces to 5 pounds, 8 ounces) at birth regardless of gestational age.

❑❑ **When teaching teenage girls about birth control, what should be recommended?**

Abstinence. The next most effective method is oral contraceptive use.

❑❑ **What is the Linea nigra?**

A dark line that extends from the umbilicus to the mons pubis and commonly appears during pregnancy.

❑❑ **What is the treatment for ankle edema in a pregnant patient?**

Frequent rest periods, foot elevation, and avoidance of constrictive clothing such as a garter or knee-high hose.

❑❑ **What are the findings in a neonate with hypoglycemia?**

Temperature instability, hypotonia, jitteriness, and seizures.

❑❑ **What are the findings in a patient with a ruptured ectopic pregnancy?**

Sharp lower abdominal pain with spotting and cramping, abdominal rigidity, rapid shallow respirations, tachycardia, and shock.

❑❑ **What does the acronym TORCH stand for?**

Infections occuring during pregnancy which can harm an embryo or fetus:
Toxoplasmosis.
Other diseases (chlamydia, group A beta hemolytic streptococcus, syphilis and varicella zoster).
Rubella.
Cytomegalovirus.
Herpes virus.

❑❑ **What are the signs and symptoms of a chlamydial infection?**

Urinary frequency, thin white vaginal or urethral discharge, and cervical inflammation.

❑❑ **What is the most prevalent sexually transmitted disease in the U.S.?**

Chlamydia.

❑❑ **What is placenta previa?**

A placenta that has an abnormally low implantation so that it encroaches on or covers the cervical os.

❑❑ **What is Ortolani's sign?**

An audible click or palpable jerk with thigh adduction confirming a congenial hip dislocation in the neonate.

❑❑ **What are the findings in a patient with pre-eclampsia?**

Hypertension, edema, proteinuria, hyperreflexia, visual disturbances, and epigastric pain.

❑❑ **What scoring system is used to assess neonatal vital functioning after delivery?**

Apgar scoring.

❑❑ **When is Apgar scoring done?**

One and 5 minutes after birth.

❑❑ **During labor, what should the minimal resting phase be between contractions?**

30 seconds.

❑❑ **What type of a diet could help a pregnant client avoid constipation and hemorrhoids?**

High fiber diet.

❑❑ **What are the findings in a patient with Trichomonas vaginalis?**

Malodorous, frothy, and greenish-gray vaginal discharge.

❒❒ What instructions should you give to a pregnant patient who has developed late decelerations?

Instruct her to lie on her right side and notify the physician immediately.

❒❒ How long do spermatozoa remain in the vagina after sexual intercourse?

72 hours.

❒❒ If a patient misses a menstrual period while taking an oral contraceptive as prescribed, what should she do?

Continue taking the contraceptive. Missed periods can occur while taking oral contraceptives.

❒❒ If a patient taking an oral contraceptive misses a dose, what should she do?

Take the pill as soon as she remembers or take 2 at the next scheduled interval and continue with the normal schedule.

❒❒ If a patient taking an oral contraceptive misses 2 consecutive days, what should she do?

Double the dose for 2 days, then resume her normal schedule; also an additional birth control method should be used for one week.

❒❒ What is a complete abortion?

When all products of conception have been expelled.

❒❒ What is polyhydramnios?

Excessive amniotic fluid (more than 2000 ml) in the third trimester.

❒❒ Describe what occurs during the transition phase of labor.

The cervix dilates to 7-10 cm and contractions usually occur 2-3 minutes apart, lasting for 60 seconds.

❒❒ What is considered a positive non-stress test?

Fewer than 2 fetal heart accelerations of at least 15 beats per minute occurring in 20 minutes.

❒❒ For what is a non-stress test used?

Assessment of fetal well-being in the pregnant patient with a prolonged pregnancy, diabetes, a history of poor pregnancy outcome, pregnancy induced hypertension, or other pregnancy related abnormalities.

❒❒ What pregnancy-related disorder is associated with painless vaginal bleeding?

Placenta previa.

❒❒ What is the treatment for abruptio placenta?

Immediate caesarian section.

❑❑ **When should breast feeding begin?**

As soon as possible, after delivery.

❑❑ **How long should a neonate stay on each breast?**

10-15 minutes.

❑❑ **When can an amniocentesis be performed?**

15-17 weeks gestation.

❑❑ **At what time is the product of conception considered a fetus?**

From the 8th week of gestation through delivery.

❑❑ **What is the definition of an incomplete abortion?**

The fetus is expelled but parts of the placenta and membrane remain in the uterus.

❑❑ **What is the first nursing action after a neonate is delivered?**

Establish an airway.

❑❑ **What is climacteric?**

The transition period during which a woman's reproductive function diminishes and gradually disappears.

❑❑ **What is lochia rubra?**

The vaginal discharge of almost pure blood that occurs during the first few days after childbirth.

❑❑ **What is lochia serosa?**

The serous vaginal discharge that occurs about 4 to 5 days after childbirth.

❑❑ **What is lochia alba?**

The final stage of lochia characterized by a white vaginal discharge of decreased blood and increased leukocytes.

❑❑ **What 3 medications may be used to prevent ophthalmia neonatorium?**

Tetracycline, silver nitrate, or erythromycin.

❑❑ **What are the findings of premenstrual syndrome?**
Abdominal distention, backache, headache, nervousness, irritability, engorged and painful breasts, restlessness, and tremors.

❒❒ **After delivery, what can be done to help stimulate uterine contractions?**

Massage the uterus.

❒❒ **What are the symptoms of respiratory distress syndrome in a neonate?**

Expiratory grunting, harsh breath sounds, and retractions.

❒❒ **What are Kegel exercises?**

Voluntary contraction and relaxation of the peroneal muscles.

❒❒ **What is the purpose of Kegel exercises during pregnancy?**

Strengthen pelvic muscles and improve urine control in the postpartum patients.

❒❒ **What are the symptoms of postpartum depression?**

Mild depression-like symptoms to an intense suicidal depressive psychosis.

❒❒ **What are the components of the Apgar score?**

Respiratory effort, heart rate, muscle tone, reflex irritability, and color.

❒❒ **What are the most common disorders of infants born to diabetic women?**

Skeletal system abnormalities and a ventricular septal defect.

❒❒ **During fetal heart monitoring, what do variable decelerations indicate?**

Umbilical cord compression or prolapse.

❒❒ **During fetal heart monitoring, what is the cause of early decelerations?**

Head compression during labor.

❒❒ **What is the best technique for assessing jaundice in a neonate?**

Blanch the skin on the forehead.

❒❒ **What position should a female be placed in when performing a pelvic exam?**

The lithotomy position.

❒❒ **What is one side effect of clomiphene citrate (Clomid)?**

Multiple births.

❒❒ **When a patient is admitted to labor and delivery in active labor, what is your first step?**

Take her vital signs and listen for fetal heart tones.

❑❑ **What is the duration of pregnancy?**

280 days or 40 weeks.

❑❑ **What is the normal sperm count?**

20 to 200 million per ml.

❑❑ **What disorder is caused by a pituitary infarction after postpartum shock and hemorrhage?**

Sheehan's syndrome.

❑❑ **What is the cause of first trimester nausea and vomiting in pregnancy?**

Rising levels of human chorionic gonadotropin.

❑❑ **How soon after delivery may a postpartum patient resume sexual intercourse?**

4-6 weeks after delivery.

❑❑ **A pregnant nurse is assigned a patient with cytomegalovirus, what should be done?**

The nurse should be reassigned to another patient.

❑❑ **What is the most common method of inducing labor after artificial rupture of membranes?**

Oxytocin (Pitocin) infusion.

❑❑ **What are telangiectatic nevi (stork bites)?**

Normal neonatal skin lesions found on the back of the neck, upper eyelids, upper lip, and bridge of the nose. They usually regress by age 2.

❑❑ **What are the most common reasons for caesarian section?**

Fetal distress, cephalopelvic disproportion, toxemia, previous caesarian birth, inadequate progress in labor, and malposition.

❑❑ **What are the complications from an amniocentesis?**

Spontaneous abortion, trauma to the fetus or placenta, premature labor, infection, and Rh sensitization of the fetus.

❑❑ **An Rh-negative primigravida has just delivered an Rh-positive infant. What medication should she receive?**

RhoGAM.

PEDIATRIC PEARLS

"Somebody BOUNCED me. I was just thinking by the side of the river...
when I received a loud BOUNCE."
Eeyore

❑❑ What is the appropriate bolus for a dehydrated child weighing 15 kg?

300 ml (20 ml/kg).

❑❑ What are the signs and symptoms of intestinal obstruction in a newborn?

Maternal polyhydramnios, abdominal distention, failure to pass meconium, and vomiting.

❑❑ Torsion of the testicles is most common in what age group?

Adolescents.

❑❑ What is the maximal amount of time a testes can remain torsed without irreversible damage being done?

4–6 hours.

❑❑ What is the most sensitive indicator of shock in children?

Tachycardia.

❑❑ What is the initial fluid bolus that should be given to children in shock?

20 ml/kg.

❑❑ What is nursemaid's elbow?

Subluxation of the radial head. During forceful retraction, some fibers of the annular ligament that encircle the radial neck become trapped between the radial head and the capitellum. On presentation, the arm is held in slight flexion and pronation.

❑❑ What is a common transport medium that can be used in an emergency for an avulsed tooth?

Milk, or the patient, if he/she is able to keep from aspirating, may place the tooth underneath the tongue.

❑❑ Why are preschool children more susceptible to acute otitis media?

Eustachian tube dysfunction is the most important factor contributing to acute otitis media. Children's shorter, more horizontal eustachian tubes may prevent adequate drainage and allow aspiration of nasopharyngeal bacteria into the middle ear particularly with URIs.

❑❑ **What are the most common extrinsic allergens that affect asthmatic children?**

Dust and dust mites.

❑❑ **Asthmatics will most likely have a family history of what?**

Asthma, allergies, or atopic dermatitis.

❑❑ **A 2-year-old patient presents with a sudden harsh cough that is worse at night, with wheezing, and rhonchi/inspiratory stridor. What is the probable diagnosis?**

Croup (also known as laryngotracheitis). This condition is usually preceded by an URI and most frequently caused by the parainfluenza virus. A barking seal cough is a characteristic of croup.

❑❑ **What age group is afflicted with the most colds per year?**

Kindergartners win the top billing with an average of 12 colds per year. Second place goes to preschoolers with 6-10 per year. School children get an average of 7 per year, and adolescents and adults average only 2-4 per year.

❑❑ **What is the duration of a common cold?**

3-10 day self limited course.

❑❑ **Which age group usually contracts croup?**

6 months to 3 years. Croup is characterized by cold symptoms, a sudden barking cough, inspiratory and expiratory stridor, and a slight fever.

❑❑ **A newborn presents with poor weight gain, steatorrhea, and a GI obstruction arising from thick meconium ileus. You order a sweat test. Why?**

The sweat test detects electrolyte concentrations in the sweat. The infant may have cystic fibrosis. Cystic fibrosis is an autosomal recessive defect affecting the exocrine glands. As a result, electrolyte concentrations increase in the sweat glands.

❑❑ **What is the classic triad of cystic fibrosis?**

1) COPD.
2) Pancreatic enzyme deficiency.
3) Abnormally high concentration of sweat electrolytes.

❑❑ **What is the most common presentation of newborns with cystic fibrosis?**

GI obstruction due to meconium ileus.

❑❑ **What is the difference between the "cough of croup" and the "cough of epiglottitis"?**

Croup has a seal like "barking" cough, while epiglottitis is accompanied by a minimal cough. Children with croup have a hoarse voice while those with epiglottitis have a muffled voice.

❑❑ **Should a 7-year-old who has never received her Hib vaccine be vaccinated now?**

No, most children are immune by the age of 5.

❑❑ **How is fetal lung maturity assessed?**

By measuring the ratio of lecithin to sphingomyelin (L/S). An L/S ratio greater than 2 and the presence of phosphatidyl glycerol verifies that the fetal lungs are mature.

❑❑ **Are aspirated foreign bodies more likely to be found in the right or left bronchus and why?**

The right bronchus because it is straighter and foreign objects are more likely to follow this path.

❑❑ **Name the most probable cause of diarrhea in a 6-month-old in day-care.**

Viral diarrhea caused by Rotavirus is the most common. Also Giardia and Cryptosporidia have recently been added to the list of day-care-associated diarrheal illnesses.

❑❑ **What is the most common cause of bacterial diarrhea?**

E. coli (enteroinvasive, enteropathogenic, enterotoxigenic).

❑❑ **Which is the most common form of acute diarrhea?**

Viral diarrhea. It is generally self limited, lasting only 1- 3 days.

❑❑ **X-rays are crucial for finding suspected swallowed foreign bodies. In kids, what physical findings can tip you off?**

Besides the child's distress, a red or scratched oropharynx, dysphagia, a high fever, or peritoneal signs may be evident. In addition, subcutaneous air suggests perforation.

❑❑ **Currant jelly stool in a child is indicative of what?**

Intussusception.

❑❑ **What is the most common cause of bowel obstruction in children under 2?**

Intussusception. Usually the terminal ileum will slide into the right colon. The cause is unknown but suspected to be due to hypertrophied lymph nodes at the junction of the ileum and colon.

❑❑ **What is the treatment for intussusception?**

A barium enema is both a diagnostic tool and curative (i.e., by reducing the intussusception). If the barium enema is unsuccessful, surgical reduction may be required.

❑❑ **What causes cerebral palsy?**

70% of the cases are idiopathic. Other causes are in utero infections, chromosomal abnormalities, or strokes. Cerebral palsy is a defect in the central nervous system that occurs prenatally, perinatally, or before the age of 3. Mental retardation occurs in 25% of patients with cerebral palsy.

❑❑ **A baby girl was born to a man who developed Huntington's chorea at the age of 44. What are her chances of developing the same disease?**

50%. Huntington's chorea is an autosomal dominant disorder that first manifests itself between the ages of 30-50. Unfortunately, this little girl can expect to become demented, amnesiac, delusional, emotionally unstable, depressed, paranoid, antisocial, and irritable if she inherits the disease. She will also develop chorea, bradykinesia, hypertonia, hyperkinesia, clonus, schizophrenia, intellectual impairment, and bowel incontinence. She will eventually die a premature death 15 years after the onset of her symptoms.

❑❑ **Why should you be especially concerned with the presence of a purpuric, petechial rash along with a febrile illness in an infant?**

Because of the possibility of Meningococcemia. Other causes include Haemophilus influenzae, Streptococcus pneumoniae, and Staphylococcus aureus.

❑❑ **A mother brings her 5-year-old son in because he was just bitten by the neighbor's dog. She is frantic because she fears he will now develop rabies. What could you tell her to calm her fears?**

The incidence of rabies in the U.S. is 0-3 cases a year. The likelihood that her son is infected is low. However, if the dog has not been vaccinated or appears ill, it should be quarantined for 10 days and observed.

❑❑ **In the U.S., what animals are most likely to be infected with the rabies virus?**

Bats, skunks, and raccoons. Dogs are the usual carriers in developing countries.

❑❑ **How should a rabies wound be treated?**

Wound care of a suspected rabies bite should include debridement and irrigation. The physician will not suture the wound, because it should remain open. This will decrease the rabies infection by 90%.

❑❑ **A 6-year-old child presents with headache, fever, malaise, and tender regional lymphadenopathy about a week after a cat bite. A tender papule develops at the site. What diagnosis should be suspected by the nurse?**

Cat-scratch disease. This condition usually develops 3 days to 6 weeks following a cat bite or scratch. The papule typically blisters and heals with eschar formation. A transient macular or vesicular rash may also develop.

❑❑ **A child has painful swollen joints along with a spiking high fever, shaking chills, signs of pericarditis, and a pale erythematous coalescing rash on the trunk, palms, and soles. Hepatosplenomegaly is found. What is the probable diagnosis?**

Systemic juvenile rheumatoid arthritis. Arthrocentesis is necessary to eliminate the possibility of septic arthritis. The rheumatoid factor and the antinuclear antibody titers usually are negative; one-fourth of patients will proceed to have joint destruction. This is the least common of the 3 types of JRA.

❑❑ **Why is surgical correction of cryptorchidism important?**

Cryptorchidism is when a testicle does not descend into the scrotum and is retained either in the abdominal cavity or in the inguinal canal. This condition can cause infertility in the affected testae and will increase the risk of cancer in that testicle. Surgical correction is required to inhibit infertility, but the procedure has no bearing on the future development of testicular cancer. Surgery must be performed before the age of 5 to preserve fertility.

❑❑ What does epididymitis in childhood suggest?

Obstructive or fistulous urinary defects. Epididymitis is rare in children.

❑❑ Testicular torsion is most common in which age group?

14-year-olds. Two-thirds of the cases occur in the second decade. The next most common group is newborns.

❑❑ T/F: Testicular torsion frequently follows a history of strenuous physical activity or occurs during sleep.

True.

❑❑ What is the definitive treatment for testicular torsion?

Bilateral orchiopexy in which the testes are surgically attached to the scrotum.

❑❑ What is the most common renal tumor in children?

Wilm's tumor. This occurs in children under 5 years of age.

❑❑ A mother is worried that her 5-year-old will get chicken pox because she was playing with her neighbor who was diagnosed with chicken pox and had crusty lesions all over his body. If this was the only day she played with the neighbor will she develop chicken pox too?

No. Chicken pox is only contagious 48 hours before the rash breaks out and until the vesicles have crusted over.

❑❑ What is the most common organism causing impetigo?

50–90% of impetigo contagiosa cases are caused by Staphylococcus aureus alone.

❑❑ A 12-year-old female comes to the physician's office complaining of intense itching in the webs between her fingers that worsens at night. On close examination you see a few small squiggly lines 1 cm x 1 mm where the patient has been scratching herself. Diagnosis?

Scabies. Scabies are due to the mite Sarcoptes scabiei var. hominis. Scabies are spread by close contact; therefore, all household contacts should also be treated.

❑❑ Tinea capitis is most commonly seen in what age group?

Children aged 4–14. This is a fungal infection of the scalp that begins as a papule around one hair shaft and then spreads to other follicles. The infection can cause the hairs to break off, leaving little black stumps and patches of alopecia. Trichophyton tonsurans is responsible for 90% of the cases. Wood's lamp examination will fluoresce only Microsporum infections, which are responsible for the remaining 10%. This is also called "ringworm of the scalp."

LPN

PEARLS OF WISDOM

Sheryl L. Gossman
William G. Gossman
Dorothy Thompson

NOTE

The intent of *LPN Pearls of Wisdom* is to serve as a study aid to improve performance on a standardized exam. It is not intended to be a source text of the knowledge base of the nursing field, or to serve as a reference in any way for the practice of clinical nursing. Neither Boston Medical Publishing Corporation, nor the editors warrant that the information in this text is complete or accurate. The reader is encouraged to verify each answer in several references. All drug use indications and dosages must be verified by the reader before administration of any compound.

Printed by Mount Auburn Press/IKON Office Solutions, Watertown, MA.

Art Director: Maryse Charette

This book was produced using Times and Symbols fonts and computer based graphics with Macintosh® computers.

ISBN: 1-58409-002-2

❐❐ **Child development: At what age are infants able to perform the following motor skills?**

1) Sit up by themselves.
2) Walk.
3) Crawl.
4) Walk up stairs.
5) Smile.
6) Hold their head up.
7) Roll over.

Answers: (1) 5–7 months, (2) 11–16 months, (3) 9–10 months, (4) 14–22 months, (5) 2 months, (6) 2–4 months, and (7) 2–6 months.

❐❐ **At what age are infants capable of the following language skills?**

1) "Mama/Dada" sounds.
2) One word.
3) Naming body parts.
4) Combine words.
5) Understandable speech.

Answers: (1) 6–10 months, (2) 9–15 months, (3) 19–25 months, (4) 17–25 months, and (5) 2–4 years.

❐❐ **At what age will a child be able to uncover a toy that is hidden by a scarf?**

9–10 months. This is called object permanence—the understanding that "out of sight" is not "out of existence."

❐❐ **Joe Montana comes to you with his 3-year-old son distressed that he can't catch a ball to save his life. You reassure Joe that children are not expected to perform that motor skill until they are what age?**

5–6 years old.

❐❐ **How many times a day should a healthy infant feed in the first 3 months of life?**

Infants should average 6–8 feedings a day. The schedule should be dictated by the infant (i.e., when he/she is hungry). By 8 months, feedings are generally only 3–4 times a day.

❐❐ **At what age may a mother switch from breast feeding or formula to whole cow's milk?**

9–12 months. Skim milk should not be given until the child is 2 years old.

❐❐ **What, if any, nutritional value does cow's milk have over breast milk?**

Cow's milk has a higher protein content than breast milk. Both have the same caloric content (20 kcal/oz). Breast milk has a higher carbohydrate concentration, a greater amount of polyunsaturated fat, and is easier for the infant to digest. And for the obvious immunological advantage, "breast is best."

❐❐ **At what age should solid foods be introduced?**

4–6 months. One food should be introduced at a time with 1–2 week intervals between the introduction of a new food. This way potential allergies can be defined.

❑❑ **How much weight should an infant gain per day in the first 2 months of life?**

15–30 gm/day. Newborns commonly lose 10% of their body weight during the first week of life due to a loss of extracellular water and a decrease in caloric intake. Healthy infants soon double their birth weight in 5 months and triple their weight in a year.

❑❑ **When do infants begin teething?**

By 6 months. They may become irritable with a decreased appetite and excessive drooling. Acetaminophen can be used to control the pain.

❑❑ **What infant immunization is most likely to cause a reaction in infants receiving standard immunizations?**

The pertussis component of the DTP. Minor reactions (local induration and pain, mild fever) occur in 75% of children who receive the vaccine. This is the most common reaction though reactions can be as severe as shock, encephalopathy, and convulsions.

❑❑ **When should toilet training be started?**

Not until at least 18 months.

❑❑ **What are the signs and symptoms of Reye's syndrome:**

The patient is usually between ages 6–11 with prior viral illness and possible use of ASA followed by intractable vomiting. Patient may be irritable, combative, or lethargic, and may complain of right upper quadrant tenderness. Seizures may occur; check for papilledema. Lab findings would include hypoglycemia and an elevated ammonia level (> 20 times normal). Bilirubin level is normal.

❑❑ **What percentage of infants have colic?**

25%. The etiology is unknown.

❑❑ **When does physiological jaundice of the newborn occur?**

2–4 days after birth. Bilirubin levels may rise up to 5–6 mg/dl.

❑❑ **Name some causes of jaundice occuring in the first day of life.**

Sepsis, congenital infections, and ABO/Rh incompatibility.

❑❑ **What is the normal pulse rate of a newborn?**

120–160 bpm.

❑❑ **Sudden Infant Death Syndrome (SIDS) is the most common cause of death for infants in the first year of life. It occurs at a rate of 2/1000, or 10,000/year. What are 6 risk factors associated with SIDS?**

1) Prematurity with low birth weight.
2) Previous episode of apnea or apparent life-threatening event (ALTE).
3) Mother is a substance abuser.
4) Family history of SIDS.
5) Male gender.
6) Low socioeconomic status.

❒❒ **At what age does SID most commonly occur?**

2 to 4 months.

❒❒ **Define failure to thrive (FTT).**

FTT is defined as infants who are below the third percentile in height or weight or whose weight is less than 80% of the ideal weight for their age. Almost all patients with FTT are under 5 years old, while the majority of children are 6–12 months old. Other disorders that are commonly confused with FTT are as follows: anorexia nervosa, bronchiectasis, cystic fibrosis, congenital heart disease, chronic renal disease, Downs syndrome, hypothyroidism, inflammatory bowel disease, juvenile rheumatoid arthritis, HIV, Hirschsprung's disease, tuberculosis, malignancy, or Turner's syndrome.

❒❒ **What is the most common cause of (FTT)?**

Poor intake is responsible for 70% of FTT cases. One third of these cases are educational problems, ranging from inaccurate knowledge of what to feed a child to over-diluting formula to "make it stretch further." While in the hospital, patients are fed a 150–200 kcal/kg/day diet (1 1/2 times their expected intake) which will correct the underlying problem if that problem is poor intake. Cases of FTT that are not due to the environment are neurological or gastrointestinal in etiology.

❒❒ **What is the prognosis for patients with FTT?**

Only one-third of patients with FTT due to environmental factors have a normal life. The remainder grow up small for their size, and the majority also have developmental, psychological, and educational deficiencies.

❒❒ **What radiological evidence would lead you to suspect child abuse?**

1) Spiral fractures, especially prior to the onset of walking.
2) Scapula or sternal fractures.
3) Chip fractures or bucket handle fractures.
4) Epiphyseal-metaphyseal rib fractures in infants.
5) Broken bones are found in 10–20% of abused children.

❒❒ **What are some other clinical findings that would lead you to suspect child abuse?**

"Accident prone" children, cigarette burns, retinal hemorrhages, subdural hematomas, head contusions in children that are pre-ambulatory, back bruises in children that can't climb, burns on the buttocks or a stocking glove distribution, and lesions in the shape of familiar objects (belts, hands).

❒❒ **How old is the average abused child?**

One-third are less than 1 year old; one-third are 1–6 years old; and one-third are over 6. Child abuse is the second highest cause of death in children aged 0–6. Premature infants are at 3 times greater a risk of being abuse.

❒❒ **What is the first sign of puberty in the male?**

Puberty in the male begins with the growth of the testes followed by thinning and pigmentation of the scrotum, growth of the penis, and lastly the development of pubic hair.

❒❒ **What is an abnormal lead level in a child?**

10 ml/dl. Symptoms of lead poisoning can include clumsiness, decreased play, lethargy, vomiting, stupor, ataxia, seizures, and coma. Chronic lead poisoning can cause behavioral and developmental problems.

❒❒ **What percentage of African-Americans are heterozygous for the sickle cell gene?**

10%. Sickle cell is also common in Greek, Turkish, Arabian, and Indian populations.

❒❒ **What commonly precipitates an aplastic crisis in a sickle cell child?**

Viral infections.

❒❒ **What organs are most commonly damaged in sickle cell patients?**

Spleen, lung, liver, kidney, skeleton, and skin.

❒❒ **An hour old premature infant presents with tachypnea, grunting, chest wall retractions, nasal flaring, and cyanosis. Diagnosis?**

Hyaline membrane disease, also known as respiratory distress syndrome of the newborn. These patients have atelectasis, intrapulmonary shunting, hypoxemia, and cyanosis.

❒❒ **What is the pathophysiology behind hyaline membrane disease?**

The lungs are poorly compliant because of a lack of sufficient surfactant. These infants are generally preterm and have not developed chemically mature lungs.

❒❒ **What percentage of children with asthma are likely to have symptoms that persist into adulthood?**

50%.

❒❒ **What is the most common cause of bronchiolitis?**

RSV.

❒❒ **What is the common age range for bronchiolitis?**

Though it may occur in patients up to age 2, bronchiolitis commonly occurs between 2–6 months, as maternal antibody to RSV is waning.

❒❒ **Define apnea.**

No respiration for > 20 seconds.

❒❒ **How long should a school-aged child receive antibiotic treatment for Strep Throat before being**

allowed to return to school?

1 day.

❑❑ **What is the most common hematological disorder in infancy?**

Iron deficiency anemia. This is generally caused by a diet poor in iron. Other causes of anemia in babies are lead poisoning and thalassemia.

❑❑ **20% of children with meningococcemia die. What is the major cause of death in these patients?**

Shock. Rapid administration of penicillin is the treatment of choice.

❑❑ **What is the most common cause of neonatal conjunctivitis?**

A trick question, as chemical conjunctivitis due to silver nitrate is most common. Chlamydia trachomatis is the most common clinically significant cause in the first 14 days with a usual incubation period of at least 5 days. Gonococcal conjunctivitis has a shorter incubation and may present as soon as 2 days.

❑❑ **What is the most common cause of tonsillitis?**

Viral (75%). Only 25% of the cases are due to ß-hemolytic streptococcus.

❑❑ **What are the indications for tonsillectomy?**

Peritonsillar abscess, airway obstruction, 7 episodes of documented streptococcal tonsillitis within 1 year, or 5 documented cases of streptococcal tonsillitis per year for 2 consecutive years.

❑❑ **Which type of agent is the most common cause of acute otitis media (AOM), bacteria or viruses?**

Bacteria—Streptococcus pneumoniae and H. influenzae are responsible for 70% of AOM.

❑❑ **What is the most common cause of croup?**

The majority of croup cases are caused by viruses, most commonly the parainfluenza virus.

❑❑ **What bone is most commonly fractured in newborns?**

The clavicle. Treatment is pinning the infants sleeve to the front of his/her shirt.

❑❑ **A mother comes to you very concerned because her 18-month-old daughter has bowlegs and she doesn't want her stigmatized as one of those children with the funny braces. What do you tell her?**

Bowlegs are caused by internal tibial torsion which spontaneously resolves by the age of 8 in 95% of children. Most likely her daughter will not have to wear braces, especially if she promises to help her daughter with a few simple leg exercises.

❑❑ **What is the most common foot deformity in the newborn?**

Calcaneovalgus foot. The infant's foot has lateral deviation of the heel, a banana-shaped sole, and an abnormally long heel chord that allows extreme dorsiflexion. The deformity occurs secondary to in utero positioning and resolves spontaneously in the large majority of cases.

❑❑ A newborn baby you are examining has kidney-shaped soles of his feet and a medial deviation of his heels. You are not able to dorsiflex his feet. What is the diagnosis?

"Club foot" or what is medically known as talipes equinovarus. Mild cases may be attributed to positioning in utero. More serious cases are due to anatomical abnormalities; like congenital convex pes valgus, this anatomical abnormality may also be associated with spina bifida.

❑❑ A 3-year-old girl is brought to your office. She is holding her right arm flexed at the elbow with her forearm pronated. She will not let you near it. Probable diagnosis?

Subluxation of the radial head (nursemaid's elbow). This injury commonly occurs when an adult pulls or jerks a child up by the arm.

❑❑ Differentiate between sprain and strain.

Sprains are stretches or incomplete tears of a ligament.

Strains are when tendons or muscles are stretched.

❑❑ When is the peak incidence of scoliosis?

Early adolescence. It is most commonly idiopathic in origin. Females are more frequently affected than males.

❑❑ What are the most common risk factors for inguinal hernias in the pediatric population?

Male gender and prematurity.

❑❑ What is the most common malignancy of childhood?

Acute lymphoblastic leukemia. Leukemia accounts for one-third of all cancers diagnosed in the pediatric population.

❑❑ What is the name for congenital aganglionic megacolon?

Hirschsprung's disease. In this disease, a portion of the distal colon lacks ganglion cells, thus impairing the normal inhibitory innervation in the myenteric plexus. This impedes coordinated relaxation, which can, in turn, cause clinical symptoms of obstruction 85% of the time after the newborn period.

❑❑ What signs and symptoms are associated with increased probability of a bacterial pathogen as a cause of diarrhea?

Fever, acute onset of multiple diarrhea stools/day, and blood in the stool.

❑❑ What is the most common intra-abdominal neoplasm in the pediatric population?

Lymphoma. Wilm's tumor is the second most common neoplasm.

❑❑ Is constipation more common in breast-fed or formula-fed infants?

Formula-fed infants. It is very rare in breast-fed infants. Treatment involves increasing the amount of fluid and/or sugar in the formula, and adding prune juice, fruits, cereal, and vegetables to the baby's diet to increase bulk.

❒❒ A new mother brings in her 3-week old infant boy because he doesn't seem to be growing and has constipation and intermittent vomiting "with such force he can almost hit the refrigerator clear across the kitchen table from where he sits." What might you expect on abdominal examination?

A small, firm, and mobile olive-shaped mass in the RUQ or epigastric area. This patient most likely has pyloric stenosis. If the stenosed pylorus cannot be palpated, then ultrasound or x-ray will reveal the defect. Treatment is pyloromyotomy.

❒❒ What is the average age of onset for pyloric stenosis?

4 weeks. The onset of pyloric stenosis is generally between the second and the fourth weeks of life; it's rarely diagnosed after 5 months.

❒❒ What is the association between prematurity and hyaline membrane disease?

The incidence of this disease is greatest in premature babies. At 29 weeks gestation, 60% of newborns will have HMD, and by 39 weeks gestation, the incidence is nearly 0%. Treatment includes trying to prevent premature birth, glucocorticoid hormones, and surfactant replacement for mothers who must deliver prematurely.

❒❒ What are some risk factors of otitis media?

Recent URI, Caucasian race, male gender, craniofacial abnormalities, Down syndrome, bottle feeding, daycare, secondhand smoke, and family history of middle ear disease.

❒❒ How common is otitis media?

Very common. By 6 months of age, 35% of children have had one episode of otitis media and by age 7, 93% of children have had one or more bouts. 39% of children have had 6 or more episodes of acute otitis media. Otitis media most commonly affects children ages 5–24 months.

❒❒ What is the most common cause of seasonal allergic rhinitis in the pediatric population?

Ragweed pollen, otherwise known as hay fever. The most common perennial allergen is house dust and house mites, followed by feathers, dander, and mold spores. Removal of the allergen, if possible, is the best treatment. Pharmacologically, sodium cromoglycate or intranasal corticosteroids are recommended.

❒❒ A 7-year-old girl with a history of strep throat 3 weeks ago presents to the physician's office complaining of joint pain "everywhere," fever, and "hard bumps" on her elbows and forearm. Probable diagnosis?

Rheumatic fever. Rheumatic fever is most common in children 5–15. It is always preceded by an infection with group A Streptococcus.

❒❒ What percent of children have heart murmurs?

50%! Only 10% of children with heart murmurs have pathological heart murmurs.

❑❑ **What are some examples of congenital heart disorders?**

Ventricular septal defects account for about 38% of all congenital heart disorders. Other disorders include atrial septal defects (18%), pulmonary valve stenosis (13%), pulmonary artery stenosis (7%), aortic valve stenosis (4%), patent ductus arteriosis (4%), and mitral valve prolapse (4%).

❑❑ **What is the most common congenital heart disease associated with Down syndrome?**

Septal defects, most commonly endocardial cushion defects (inflow ventricular septal defects that have associated abnormalities of the tricuspid and mitral valves).

❑❑ **Do not skip this question. Make a real attempt to answer it! Name 8 clinical presentations of pediatric heart disease.**

1) Cyanosis.
2) CHF.
3) Pathologic murmur.
4) Cardiogenic shock.
5) HTN.
6) Tachyarrhythmias.
7) Abnormal pulses.
8) Syncope.

❑❑ **Describe 2 nursing measures which can be implemented in the acute treatment of Tetralogy of Fallot (TOF).**

Positioning: Place in knee-chest position. Keep patient unstimulated (i.e., upright on lap in parent's arms).

Oxygenation: Deliver high FiO2.

❑❑ **Coarctation of the aorta is associated with a narrowing of the aortic arch. Where is the narrowing located?**

Just distal to the origin of the left subclavian. This results in hypertensive upper extremities and normotensive lower extremities.

❑❑ **What are the 4 defects in the Tetralogy of Fallot?**

1) Pulmonary stenosis.
2) Right ventricular hypertrophy.
3) Ventricular septal defect.
4) Dextroposition of the aorta.

❑❑ **By what age will a child reach half his/her adult height?**

2 years. However, by 2 years, most children are only 20% of their adult weight.

❑❑ **A 4-year-old girl is brought to the office with a history of high fever for 4 days but no other clinical symptoms. Her fever subsides and macular or maculopapular rash begins on the trunk and spreads peripherally. This rash lasts about 1 day. Diagnosis?**

Roseola infantum (exanthem subitum).

❑❑ A 4-year-old boy is brought to the office with red cheeks, a low grade fever, and a maculopapular rash that began on his arms and spread to his trunk and legs. The rash has a lacy reticular pattern. Dad says the rash has come and gone for the past 2 weeks. Diagnosis?

Erythema infectiosum, also known as fifth's disease or "slapped cheek disease." The patient may also have constitutional symptoms, such as pharyngitis, headache, myalgia, coryza, or gastrointestinal problems.

❑❑ What is the most common cause of stomatitis in 1-3-year-olds?

Acute herpetic gingivostomatitis caused by the herpes simplex virus.

❑❑ A 5-year-old unimunized girl is brought to the clinic. Mom says 6 days ago her child had malaise, cough, coryza, photophobia, conjunctivitis, and a mild fever. 4 days ago, her daughter had small grayish-white dots the size of grains of sand on her buccal mucosa. 2 days ago, her fever climbed to 102°F, and she developed a morbilliform rash that began on the head and has now spread to the rest of her body. Probable diagnosis?

Measles.

❑❑ Where are Koplik spots most commonly found?

Opposite the lower molars on the buccal mucosa. They can be as small as grains of sand and are commonly grayish-white with a red areolae. They occasionally bleed.

❑❑ When is the risk of congenital defects due to maternal rubella infection greatest?

In the first few months of gestation. During months 1–3, there is a 30–60% risk of congenital defects. By the fourth month, the risk is only 10%. By 5–9 months, there is a rare chance that the child may have a defect. Congenital rubella can cause deafness, glaucoma, cataracts, retardation, and congenital heart defects.

❑❑ Of all the diaper rashes babies get, how can you distinguish candidal diaper dermatitis from just a local irritation easily treated with A&D ointment?

Babies with candidal dermatitis will have satellite lesions not located in the groin area. Otherwise, this rash presents as a large, red confluent vesiculopustular plaque with a clearly demarcated border. Treatment is with topical antifungals.

❑❑ Your own child abruptly began vomiting and complaining of a sore throat and chills 4 days ago. Two days ago, her fever peaked. Yesterday, she developed an erythematous, finely-punctuated sandpaper-like rash that started on the trunk and spread outward. The lesions blanched with pressure and you noticed increased erythema in the folds of the skin. In addition to a rash, she had a strawberry tongue. Yesterday, the rash disappeared and the skin desquamated. Probable diagnosis?

Scarlet fever.

❑❑ What is the major cause of fever in an infant 0–3 months of age?

Virus (95%).

❏❏ **Febrile seizures occur when the patient's temperature does what?**

Rises rapidly. Febrile seizures are more closely related to the rapid rise in temperature than in the actual temperature reached. They occur between 6 months and 6 years of age and are thus labeled if they occur within the context of a febrile illness, last less than 15 minutes, and are tonic-clonic generalized and simple. They must have no focal neurological defects and be present in a patient with no prior neurological disorders.

❏❏ **How long must a continuous seizure last to be defined as status epilepticus?**

30 minutes.

❏❏ **What is the initial drug of choice for a patient in status epilepticus?**

Diazepam (Valium) 0.3 mg/kg at 1 mg/min. This dose can be repeated as needed up to 2.6 mg/kg.

❏❏ **What should the urine output of a pediatric patient be maintained at?**

1–2 ml/kg/h.

❏❏ **Which is a more common cause of dysuria among female pediatric patients, UTI or vulvovaginitis?**

Vulvovaginitis.

❏❏ **What percentage of infants born to HIV-infected mothers will have the HIV infection?**

30–50%.

❏❏ **In what percentage of cases of child sexual abuse is the abuser known by the child?**

90%.

❏❏ **In what percentage of cases of child abuse is the mother also abused?**

50%.

❏❏ **What are the most common ages for physical abuse in children?**

Two-thirds of physically abused children are under the age of 3, and one-third are under the age of 6 months.

❏❏ **Simple repetitive reactions like nail biting, thumb sucking, masturbation, or temper tantrums are manifestations of what psychological reaction in infancy?**

Adjustment reactions. These are responses to separation from the caregiver.

❏❏ **What is the most common cause of referral to child psychiatrists?**

Attention Deficit Hyperactivity Disorder. For those of you not paying attention, the answer again was Attention Deficit Hyperactivity Disorder. ADHD accounts for 30–50% of child psychiatric outpatients.

❑❑ **What are the side effects of methylphenidate (Ritalin)?**

Methylphenidate (Ritalin) is a psychostimulant used to treat ADHD. Side effects include depression, headache, hypertension, insomnia, and abdominal pain.

❑❑ **By what age do most children stop wetting their beds?**

By age 4. Bed wetting after this age is considered enuresis.

❑❑ **What is the medical treatment for idiopathic enuresis?**

Desmopressin (DDAVP) nose drops or imipramine (Tofranil). Most cases eventually resolve spontaneously.

❑❑ **What disorder should a 12-year-old who snorts and shouts obscenities uncontrollably be evaluated for?**

Gilles de la Tourette syndrome. It develops in childhood with facial twitches, uncontrollable arm movements, and tics. The condition worsens in adolescence.

❑❑ **A 6-year-old boy consistently wets his pants. You tell the mother to reward dry periods with treats and praise. This will help reinforce desired behavior. What kind of conditioning is this?**

Positive operant conditioning. This principle was defined by Pavlov.

❑❑ **At what age will a child understand concrete operations as defined by Piaget?**

6–12 years. By this age a child is able to tell that a line of 5 pennies all touching is equal to those same 5 pennies spread out into a much longer line.

❑❑ **Separation anxiety has an average onset of what age?**

Age 9. These children fear leaving home, sleep, being alone, going to school, and losing their parents. 75% develop somatic complaints in order to avoid attending school.

❑❑ **By what age are children aware of their own sex?**

18 months. By age 2–3, a child can answer the question as to whether he/she is a boy or a girl.

❑❑ **What is appropriate preventive immunization for a child with sickle cell anemia?**

Children with the sickle cell trait should receive all of the immunizations required of their age group plus Haemophilus B conjugate, Hepatitis B immunization, and a pneumococcal vaccine. These children should also take folic acid supplements and prophylactic penicillin V until the age of 3.

❑❑ **Which strain of influenza is more common in adults and which strain is more common in children?**

Adults: Influenza A. Children: Influenza B.

❒❒ **A complication of central sleep apnea in a child is:**

SIDS. Affected children develop morning cyanosis. However, children can be treated with theophylline.

❒❒ **What is the most common cause of death among children between 1–12 month(s) old?**

Sudden infant death syndrome (SIDS).

❒❒ **At what age do umbilical hernias typically close?**

2.

❒❒ **What type of defect produces diminished pulses in the lower extremities of a pediatric patient?**

Coarctation of the aorta.

❒❒ **What are the signs and symptoms of aortic stenosis in a child?**

Exercise intolerance, chest pain, and a systolic ejection click with a crescendo/decrescendo murmur radiating to the neck with a suprasternal thrill. No cyanosis!

❒❒ **What are the signs of left-sided heart failure in an infant?**

Increased respiratory rate, shortness of breath, and sweating during feeding.

❒❒ **What is the most common cause of viral pneumonia in the pediatric client?**

Respiratory syncytial virus (RSV).

❒❒ **How do steroids function in the treatment of asthma?**

Steroids decrease inflammation.

❒❒ **What 2 viral illnesses are prodromes for Reye's syndrome?**

Varicella (chicken pox) and influenzae B.

❒❒ **What are the signs and symptoms of Reye's syndrome?**

Irritability, combativeness, and lethargy, right upper quadrant tenderness, history of influenzae B or recent chicken pox, papilledema, hypoglycemia, and seizures. Lab results reveal hypoglycemia, an ammonia level greater than 20 times normal, and a bilirubin level that is normal.

❒❒ **What is the most common viral gastroenteritis in children?**

Rotavirus.

❒❒ **A child presents with bluish discoloration of the gingiva. What diagnosis should you suspect?**

Chronic lead poisoning. Expect the erythrocyte protoporphyrin level to be elevated in this condition.

❑❑ **What is the most common dysrhythmia in a child?**

Paroxysmal atrial tachycardia.

❑❑ **What is the most common cause of pelvic pain in adolescent females?**

An ovarian cyst.

❑❑ **How many days after a measles vaccine could a fever and a rash be expected to develop?**

7–10 days.

❑❑ **Describe a typical client with intussusception.**

Intussusception usually occurs in children of ages 3 months to 2 years. The majority are 5-10 months old, and it is more common in boys. The area of the ileocecal valve is typically the source of the problem.

❑❑ **Describe the symptoms and signs of varicella (chicken pox).**

The onset of varicella rash is 1–2 days after prodromal symptoms of slight malaise, anorexia, and fever. The rash begins on the trunk and scalp, appearing as faint macules and later becoming vesicles.

❑❑ **How is the normal systolic blood pressure (SBP) for pediatric patients (toddlers and up) calculated?**

Average SBP (mm Hg) = (patient's Age x 2) + 90.
Low normal limit SBP (mm Hg) = (patient's Age x 2) + 70.
SBP for a term newborn is about 60 mm Hg.

❑❑ **What is the most common cause of abdominal pain in children?**

Constipation.

❑❑ **What is the most common cause of an intestinal obstruction in the patient under 2 years of age?**

Intussusception.

❑❑ **What are the classic findings of shaken baby syndrome?**

1) Failure to thrive.
2) Lethargy.
3) Seizures.
4) Retinal hemorrhages.
5) CT may show subarachnoid hemorrhage or subdural hematoma from torn bridging veins.

❑❑ **Newborns should stop losing weight how many days after birth?**

About 6 days.

❑❑ **What is the difference between vomiting and regurgitation?**

Very little once it's on you! Vomiting is caused by forceful diaphragmatic and abdominal muscle contraction. Regurgitation occurs without effort.

❑❑ **Is regurgitation dangerous in an otherwise thriving neonate?**

No. However, it can be dangerous for newborns with failure to thrive or respiratory problems, and it may be associated with chronic aspiration.

❑❑ **Projectile vomiting in the neonate is often associated with pyloric stenosis. When this is the case, such vomiting becomes a prominent sign at what age?**

2–3 weeks.

❑❑ **What is the normal blood pressure in a newborn?**

60 mmHg.

❑❑ **What vaccinations are given during the first year of life?**

Polio, DPT, and Haemophilus Influenza. Some pediatricians are also recommending Hepatitis B and chicken pox.

❑❑ **When is an infant usually ready for weaning?**

Although this behavior is highly individual, when the infant beings to show interest in trying different solid foods, is breast feeding less, and eating on a regular schedule, it is usually a good time to try weaning.

❑❑ **At what age can an infant generally hold her bottle, sit without support, and begin to imitate verbal expressions?**

Approximately 9 months of age.

❑❑ **What is the muscle of choice for an injection in a 2-month-old?**

Vastus lateralis.

❑❑ **By what route is a DPT immunization administered at 2 months?**

Deep IM injection

❑❑ **At what age is a small pox vaccine routinely given?**

The smallpox vaccine is no longer routinely given.

❑❑ **What teaching should you give a parent following the administration of the DPT vaccine?**

Potential side effects of the vaccine and how to treat them. Routine administration of acetaminophen every 4 hours for 24-36 hours after an injection is often recommended.

❑❑ **What are some of the common side effects of the DPT vaccine?**

Fever, irritability, redness, and soreness at the site.

❑❑ When would the parent expect to see a fever after the administration of the DPT vaccine and how should it be treated?

12-24 hours. Treat with acetaminophen.

❑❑ The parent complains that her 6-month-old infant will not eat solid foods. What suggestions could you give for feeding?

Offer formula or breast milk first, then try solid foods before the child is full. Offer reassurance that infants are not used to the texture of food and may not know how to handle it.

❑❑ At the age of 1 month, what developmental tasks should you be looking for?

Able to lift head and move it side to side when lying prone, and turning towards sound.

❑❑ What developmental tasks would you expect a 4-month-old to perform?

Hold a rattle, turns from side to back, responds to stimulation with a smile, holds head erect when sitting, and able to take objects from hand to mouth.

❑❑ Following a DPT vaccine, how high should a parent allow the temperature to rise before calling the physician?

Once the fever reaches 102 degrees, the physician should be notified.

❑❑ Why is it not safe to leave an infant with a propped up bottle of formula or juice throughout the night?

The chance of choking is increased along with the development of dental caries at an early age.

❑❑ What does the Denver Developmental Screening Test (DDST) measure?

The child's social and physical abilities.

❑❑ At what age can an infant sit alone while leaning foreword using the hands for support?

7 months.

❑❑ At what age does and infant learn to crawl?

10 months.

❑❑ At about what age does an infant learn to walk?

12 months.

❑❑ By what age should the infant be able to sit well unsupported?

8 months.

❑❑ **At what age should a child be able to ride a tricycle?**

Age 3.

❑❑ **What is the developmental task of toddlerhood according to Erikson?**

Acquiring a sense of autonomy while overcoming a sense of doubt and shame.

❑❑ **Because of the toddler's quest for autonomy, what behavior is typical of this age?**

Negativism, doing the opposite of what is desired from them, exploration, and wanting to do things on their own.

❑❑ **A parent asks you how she should discipline her 3-year-old. What teaching could you give the parent?**

Teach the parent about rules and limit setting, calling attention to unacceptable behavior, and praising when good behavior is demonstrated. Physical punishment is not recommended and reasoning with the child at this age is not appropriate.

❑❑ **What is an important subject to teach the parents when dealing with a toddler in the home?**

Safety issues and how to childproof the home.

❑❑ **According to Piaget, when does the concept of object permanence develop in the child?**

Age 6-9 months.

❑❑ **What is one of the reasons a 2-year-old child is afraid of the dark according to Piaget?**

The concept of animism where the child attributes human qualities to inanimate objects.

❑❑ **What is Piaget's theory of conservationism?**

Seen in school age children, it is the understanding that objects remain the same even when their form and shape change.

❑❑ **How much milk should a 15-month-old receive daily?**

2-3 cups per day.

❑❑ **When instilling ear drops in the toddler, what direction should you pull the ear lobe?**

Pull the earlobe down and back to help straighten out the ear canal.

❑❑ **When a toddler is uncooperative during an exam, what should you try first?**

Ask the parent to assist. The child's uncooperative behavior is usually due to fear and asking the parent to help may put the child more at ease.

❑❑ **How often should a toddler's teeth be brushed?**

After every meal and at bedtime by the adult. A child of this age does not have the motor skills to do a good enough job.

❑❑ **Why is it usually not helpful for you to ask a toddler if he is in pain?**

The toddler may not understand the nature of the pain and may not be able to adequately communicate its location or severity. Instead look for physical clues such as guarding, irritability, and crying.

❑❑ **What is the most common reason why a toddler is not able to be potty trained?**

The toddler is not developmentally ready.

❑❑ **Children are usually farsighted until what age?**

Age 7.

❑❑ **The parents of a toddler complains that their child will only eat peanut butter and jelly sandwiches and crackers. What should you advise the parents?**

Allow the child to eat what he wants (within reason) and do not force other foods on him. Extreme food preferences are common at this age and will eventually fade. So, peanut butter and jelly for breakfast is okay for now.

❑❑ **The parent of a 4-year-old is concerned because she is always moving, always active, always running and falling down, and always dropping things. Should this mother be concerned?**

Most likely no. Preschoolers are very energetic and their underdeveloped gross motor skills cause them to have mishaps easily.

❑❑ **A patient tells you that her 4-year-old is very picky with his food and refuses to finish meals. What teaching could you do with this client?**

Explain that it is important to allow the 4-year-old to make some decisions on his own. Allowing him to choose his foods (within limits) and not forcing him to finish meals is acceptable and will avoid confrontations at mealtime. Limit setting as to the amount of snacks and sweets, before and after meals should also be discussed if that is a problem.

❑❑ **What types of games are best for preschoolers?**

Since preschoolers are active, games that involve gross motor activity and lots of movement are preferable.

❑❑ **Research has shown that childhood accidents are most likely to occur in what types of situations?**

Times of stress and change, new situations, multiple sibling homes (because the parent is distracted), and low socio-economic status.

❑❑ **What home rules can make bedtime less of a battle for the preschooler and parent?**

An established bedtime, an established bedtime routine, and limit setting when it comes to following these rules.

❑❑ **What is the purpose of giving the preschool child a play syringe and doll after receiving an**

injection?

To allow the child to feel she has regained control of the situation and to allow the child to role play and act out her fears.

❑❑ **Why is it best to tell the preschool child that an injection will hurt?**

The child understands that the injection will hurt. Lying will only decrease credibility and trust with the child.

❑❑ **At what age should parents allow their child to brush his own teeth?**

Age 7.

❑❑ **What is one of the most powerful types of teaching that can be done with the preschool age child?**

Learning by example. Preschoolers observe behavior and often imitate adults.

❑❑ **How can you test the visual acuity of a preschooler?**

Use Allen picture cards or some similar testing tool, which uses pictures rather than words to test visual acuity.

❑❑ **What are the Ishihara plates used for in visual testing?**

They test for color blindness.

❑❑ **How do preschool age children often view illness?**

As a punishment. At this age children often do not separate reality from fantasy and they may view the illness as punishment for something they did.

❑❑ **At about what age does a child develop a "best friend?"**

About age 9 or 10.

❑❑ **During middle and late childhood, what is Erikson's theory of psycosocial development called?**

Industry vs. inferiority. The child is trying to master skills to create and complete projects.

❑❑ **According to Kohlberg, when a child begins to identify behaviors that are pleasing to others, he is displaying which level of moral development?**

Conventional morality.

❑❑ **When charting a child's growth and development, what percentile is considered normal?**

Anything between the 5th and 95th percentile.

❑❑ **Approximately how many calories per day does the school age child require?**

2,400 calories per day.

❐❐ **Between ages 7 and 11, a child will often become compulsive about collecting things. This is an example of what cognitive ability?**

Concrete operations where the child learns to manipulate and classify objects.

❐❐ **What immunizations are recommended for children between ages 4 and 6 years?**

DPT booster, oral polio vaccine, and measles-mumps-rubella.

❐❐ **You examine a 6-year-old and find enlarged tonsils that are not red or inflamed. What should you do?**

Nothing. Lymph tissue is often enlarged until the age of 6 to 7 years and then it slowly atrophies. There is no need for concern unless infection is present.

❐❐ **What is the most common cause of accidental injury between the ages of 6 to 12 years?**

Motor vehicle accidents.

❐❐ **What are some of the other major causes of accidental injury and death in school age children?**

Drowning, burns, and firearms.

❐❐ **Do children over the age of 15 need any further immunizations?**

Only a combined tetanus toxoid and diphtheria booster every 10 years into adulthood is required.

❐❐ **According to Piaget, what phase of cognitive development is the adolescent going through?**

Dealing with abstract possibilities.

❐❐ **According to Kohlberg, what level of moral reasoning is the adolescent going through?**

The conventional level (stage 3) where moral reasoning is based on the approval of others.

❐❐ **Why is it important for the adolescent girl not to view menstruation as painful or debilitating?**

It is important for the adolescent to have a positive self image and it is important for her to understand that menstruation is normal and will not inhibit her activities.

❐❐ **You are examining an 8th grader and have him bend forward from the waist with his back parallel to the floor. What are you looking for?**

Idiopathic scoliosis.

❐❐ **In primary dysmenorrhea, what is the physiological cause of cramps, backaches, and nausea?**

The release of prostaglandins. The use of prostaglandin inhibitors, such as ibuprofen, usually relieves the symptoms.

❑❑ What important teaching should you do with an adolescent female who wishes to begin using tampons?

The prevention of toxic shock syndrome by changing tampons frequently.

❑❑ Why do adolescents spend a great deal of time worrying about their personal appearance?

Adolescence is a time of integrating their physical changes into their own self concept. Their appearance is important to them as they develop their identity.

❑❑ What can you suggest to the parent to help relieve the itching associated with chicken pox in their child?

Calamine lotion, oral antihistamines such as diphenhydramine (Benadryl), or a paste made of baking soda and water applied to the skin.

❑❑ What is the cause of ringworm?

Ringworm is caused by a fungus.

❑❑ What is the treatment for Ringworm?

A topical antifungal agent such as griseofulvin (Grisactin) may be ordered by the physician.

❑❑ What is an important aspect of teaching related to the administration of anti-fungal agents?

Long-term use is necessary to prevent further infection of the fungus. Anti-fungal agents bind to the keratin in the skin and prevent infection, but as the skin sheds, the new cells are left unprotected from the fungus.

❑❑ What is pediculosis capitus?

Head lice.

❑❑ How is head lice transmitted?

Close contact with infested clothing, combs, brushes, towels, and infected persons.

❑❑ How are pinworms transmitted?

Usually through hand contact with the egg, which is then transferred to the child's mouth.

❑❑ What is the primary focus in the prevention of skin infections when caring for the child with chicken pox?

To prevent itching, which can introduce organisms into the lesions and cause infection.

❑❑ What over the counter medication is contraindicated in the child with hemophilia and why?

Acetylsalicylic acid (Aspirin) because it inhibits platelet congregation.

❒❒ **What should be done when a child with hemophilia receives a cut?**

Cleanse the area and apply gentle pressure while immobilizing and elevating the affected area. Cold applications may also help.

❒❒ **Why should sexually active adolescent girls not receive the measles vaccine?**

If she becomes pregnant up to 3 months after receiving the vaccine, there is a considerable risk for fetal deformity.

❒❒ **A parent is concerned with how best to prepare her 5-year-old for the first day of school. What suggestions could the nurse give?**

Have the child visit the school and meet with the teacher to diminish the fear of the unknown.

❒❒ **When a client is diagnosed with a sexually transmitted disease, what is an important responsibility for the public health nurse?**

Identifying all previous sexual contacts with the patient and urge them to get treatment.

❒❒ **What is a common cause of unhappiness for a child first entering school?**

Feeling of insecurity related to loss of the familiar home environment.

❒❒ **What are the most common symptoms of mononucleosis?**

Fatigue, fever, sore throat, lymph node enlargement, and spleen enlargement.

❒❒ **Why are the food requirements for the school age child less than that of adolescents or toddlers?**

The growth rate is slower during this period as compared to adolescence and toddler-hood.

❒❒ **Which gender goes through adolescence at an earlier age?**

Females go through adolescence 1-2 years earlier than males.

❒❒ **Following a tonsillectomy and adenoidectomy (T&A), what position should a child be placed in and why?**

Side lying or prone to prevent the risk of aspiration.

❒❒ **Following a T&A how long should a child be kept NPO?**

Until the child is fully alert.

❒❒ **Why is coughing contraindicated following a T&A?**

It could promote bleeding.

❒❒ **What would be an indication of possible bleeding following a T&A?**

Drooling of bright red blood or frequent swallowing.

❑❑ What is usually one of the most common times for hemorrhage following a T&A after discharge?

Approximately 10 days after surgery when the tissue where the tonsils were located starts to loosen.

❑❑ A 3-month-old child has been diagnosed with Sudden Infant Death Syndrome (SIDS). How can you aid in the grieving process?

Allow the parents to see the child (this will help begin the grieving process), education regarding SIDS, information concerning support groups, and reassurances that the parents were not responsible are helpful.

❑❑ When would be the best time for the community health nurse to visit the parent of a child who died from SIDS?

As soon after the death as possible to help arrange for resources to help deal with the death.

❑❑ What is the cause of SIDS?

There is no one generally accepted cause, only theories.

❑❑ A child is admitted to the ED with a foreign body aspiration of a peanut. Why are peanuts so dangerous when aspirated?

They swell when wet causing further airway obstruction, and the peanut oils are irritating to the lungs.

❑❑ Following a bronchoscopy, what should you be assessing the patient for?

Respiratory distress caused by laryngeal edema and airway obstruction.

❑❑ How long does it take for brain death to occur if the oxygen supply is cut off?

4-6 minutes.

❑❑ What are the signs that a child is choking?

Inability to speak, cyanotic color, and collapse.

❑❑ What types of foods are easily aspirated in the young child?

Generally round or cylindrical objects such as hard candy, nuts, and hot dogs.

❑❑ Why is it important for a child to come back to the physician for an ear re-check after finishing a course of antibiotics for otitis media?

To determine if the antibiotic therapy was effective in treating the infection.

❑❑ What are the symptoms of acute otitis media?

Rhinorrhea, fever, cough, pulling at ears, ear pain, and a red bulging tympanic membrane.

❑❑ **What is one way to help prevent otitis media in an infant?**

Holding the infant upright when feeding helps prevent pooling of formula in the pharyngeal growth area.

❑❑ **Why are children more prone to ear infections that adults?**

The eustachian tubes are short and lie in a more horizontal position, allowing for secretions to travel into the middle ear easily.

❑❑ **What is the purpose of tympanostomy tubes?**

They are inserted in a child with chronic ear infections to allow ventilation into the middle ear and facilitate drainage.

❑❑ **When are tympanostomy tubes removed?**

They usually fall out on their own within 6 months.

❑❑ **What teaching should you give in regards to getting a child's ears wet after insertion of tympanostomy tubes?**

Plugs need to be placed in the child's ears if there is any chance of getting wet. This prevents water from leaking into the middle ear via the tubes.

❑❑ **A child is brought into the ED with an acute asthma attack. After a short time, you no longer hear wheezing. Why should you be concerned?**

The child's condition could have worsened and the absence of wheezing could indicate that air is not being moved through the lungs. Epinephrine should be administered.

❑❑ **What is a typical side effect of epinephrine?**

Tremors, increased heart rate, and nervousness.

❑❑ **What are some of the causes of asthma?**

A reaction of the airway to external or internal stimuli. This can include allergens, stress, anxiety, and exercise.

❑❑ **What are some of the side effects of aminophylline?**

Vomiting, headache, nervousness and irritability.

❑❑ **What are some of the signs and symptoms of aminophylline toxicity?**

Dysrrhythmias, seizures, and hypotension.

❑❑ **What is cromolyn sodium used for and how does it work?**

It is used to prevent the onset of asthma attacks by preventing histamine release. It acts locally on the mast cells by preventing a reaction to allergens.

❑❑ Antibiotics are ordered for a child 3 times a day while in the hospital. Should the doses be split equally throughout the day, or given only during waking hours.

Antibiotics should be given at equal intervals to maintain a therapeutic blood level. The child should be woken if necessary to maintain this schedule unless the physician orders otherwise.

❑❑ What is the purpose of pancreatic enzymes when given to a child with cystic fibrosis?

To aid in the digestion and absorption of nutrients normally done by the child's own pancreatic enzymes. Cystic fibrosis impairs the normal release of the child's own enzymes.

❑❑ What is important for the parent of a child with cystic fibrosis to know about their care during the summer months?

Salt loss through the sweat glands increases with sweating and usually requires replacement with salt tablets to maintain sodium balance.

❑❑ What causes cystic fibrosis?

An autosomal recessive trait inherited from both parents.

❑❑ What physiological problems occur as a result of cystic fibrosis?

It is a dysfunction with the body's mucous producing exocrine glands which results in thick, sticky mucous which clogs airways, causes infection, and prevents the adequate digestion of food.

❑❑ You find a child that is unconscious. What should you do first?

Assess level of consciousness by shaking gently and calling to the child.

❑❑ What is the proper hand technique for chest compressions in an infant?

Using 2 fingertips at the nipple line.

❑❑ What is the proper hand technique for chest compressions in a child?

Two finger's-breadth above the sternal notch using the heel of one hand.

❑❑ What should be the rate of chest compressions in a child?

80-100.

❑❑ Where is the best location to check for a pulse during CPR in an infant?

The brachial pulse in the inside portion of the upper arm.

❑❑ What is the best location for checking the pulse during CPR in a child?

The carotid.

❑❑ What should be the depth of chest compressions in a child?

1 to 1.5 inches.

❑❑ **An infant is choking. You open the mouth and see nothing. Should a finger sweep be performed?**

No. Blind finger sweeps are contraindicated in the infant because it could push an object further back into the throat.

❑❑ **At what age should abdominal thrusts not be used?**

One year of age and under due to the risk of organ damage.

❑❑ **How should you hold an infant when delivering back blows?**

Face down with the head lower than the trunk.

❑❑ **Describe some of the clinical signs of low cardiac output in a child.**

Cyanosis, weakness, pale/cool extremities, thready pulse, delayed capillary refill, and altered level of consciousness.

❑❑ **After open-heart surgery on their child, you teach the parents about subacute bacterial endocarditis precautions. What does this entail?**

Receiving IV antibiotics prior to any invasive procedure including dental procedures and maintaining good dental health.

❑❑ **When is clubbing of the fingers seen in children?**

In disorders that cause chronic hypoxia. Tissue changes in the fingers as the body attempts to improve blood supply causes the clubbing.

❑❑ **What important teaching needs to be done with the parents of a child on digoxin (Lanoxin)?**

Signs and symptoms of toxicity and keeping the medicine out of the reach of children.

❑❑ **When preparing a child for a procedure psychologically, at what age do they become able to understand basic concepts that may help them understand what they are about to under go?**

Usually preschool age. Infants and toddlers are still too young to understand.

❑❑ **After a cardiac catheterization, what assessment should you give the highest priority?**

Assessing the involved and uninvolved extremities for pulse, color, temperature, and capillary refill.

❑❑ **How does Sickle-Cell Anemia affect blood cells?**

Blood cells are sickle shaped causing difficulty in moving through capillaries.

❑❑ **If an infant with sickle cell assumes a side lying position with the knees flexed, what should you assess for?**

Evidence of abdominal pain. Since the infant cannot communicate, physical behavior may alert you to signs of discomfort.

❒❒ **What is the cause of sickle-cell disease?**

It is an autosomal recessive disorder, meaning that if both parents have the trait, then the child has a 25% chance of having the trait and a 50% chance of having the disease.

❒❒ **What is an important basic principle that should be taught to the parents of a sickle cell child?**

Keep the child well hydrated. This will help prevent the cells from backing up in the smaller capillaries.

❒❒ **What is leukemia?**

A neoplastic disorder of the bone marrow that causes the overproduction of immature white blood cells.

❒❒ **What causes a child with leukemia to bleed and bruise easily?**

A decreased amount of platelets due to the decreased production of megakaryocytes from which platelets are derived.

❒❒ **What is the major cause of death in a child with leukemia?**

Infection caused by the inability of the body to fight off pathogens due the lack of mature white blood cells.

❒❒ **What causes anemia and increased bleeding in a child suffering from leukemia?**

The bone marrow overproduces white blood cells at the expense of producing red blood cells and platelets.

❒❒ **What is the most common site for bone marrow aspiration in children?**

Posterior iliac crest.

❒❒ **The child with leukemia is prescribed mercaptopurine (Purinethol). What is the purpose of this drug?**

It is an antimetabolite that interferes with the normal cell growth and metabolism of cancer cells.

❒❒ **What are some of the signs and symptoms of mercaptopurine toxicity?**

Nausea, vomiting, diarrhea, anorexia, and low blood counts due to suppression of the bone marrow.

❒❒ **What special precautions would you implement for a child with a low granulocyte count following chemotherapy?**

A private room, limited visitors, and prevention of exposure to any type of infection due to the body's limited defense to fight off infection.

❒❒ **Why is allopurinol (Zyloprim) often given after a course of chemotherapy?**

The destruction of cells produce large amounts of uric acid, which the kidneys may not be able to eliminate, leading to renal failure. This drug helps to prevent the build up of uric acid.

❒❒ **Prior to any course of chemotherapy, what lab tests are important and why?**

A complete blood count to get a baseline cell count. Chemotherapy often causes anemia and low white blood cells and platelets. If these conditions are already present the physician may decide to postpone chemotherapy.

❒❒ **To help others deal with death, most agree that as a nurse, you should have already worked out what feelings of your own?**

You must have already examined your own personal beliefs of death and dying.

❒❒ **How should you respond if a terminally ill child asks if he is going to die?**

Honestly. Most children can sense when they are severely ill. Being honest and helping them prepare for death will help them feel less isolated.

❒❒ **What lab test will be abnormal in a child with hemophilia?**

PTT.

❒❒ **When a drug is administered via the spinal column, what route is this called?**

Intrathecal.

❒❒ **Is it contraindicated for a child with hemophilia to play sports?**

No. There are sports that involve minimal contact, such as swimming. It is healthy for the child to be involved in some sort of physical activity.

❒❒ **What is a common parental reaction related to a child with a chronic illness?**

Overprotection of the child.

❒❒ **How is hemophilia transmitted?**

It is a sex linked trait that is genetically passed on.

❒❒ **Why are most hemophiliacs male?**

It is a sex linked trait passed on the X chromosome. Therefore, females need the trait to be present on both X chromosomes to have the disease, while males need only to have one. Females with the disease trait on one X chromosome are considered carriers of the disease.

❒❒ **What teaching should be included in the long-term goals for a child who has hemophilia?**

Prevention of injury and the correct treatment when injury occurs.

❒❒ **What is a hemarthrosis?**

Bleeding into the joints.

❑❑ **What are some of the symptoms of a hemarthrosis?**

Pain and tenderness in the joint, and restricted movement. Continued bleeding results in a hot, swollen joint that is immobile.

❑❑ **Why are hemophiliacs at a high risk for contracting AIDS?**

The clotting factors are derived from large pools of donated plasma, therefore the exposure is high due to many different blood donors. With the improved blood screening process and the manufacturing of synthetic factor, the risk of AIDS contraction for hemophiliacs is lower today.

❑❑ **For a toddler with hemophilia, what special teaching should be done with the parents?**

Methods for preventing injury in the child, such as protective padding for joints and close monitoring of the child's activity.

❑❑ **For a child who receives human factor, what other diseases besides AIDS are they at risk for?**

Any disease transmitted by the blood, such as hepatitis.

❑❑ **Why are intramuscular injections kept to a minimum for a child with Leukemia and Hemophilia?**

Both are prone to abnormal bleeding, but for different reasons.

❑❑ **You see a parent using a toothbrush on her child who has leukemia and instruct her to stop. Why?**

Toothbrushes are considered too rough when a child is prone to gum bleeding. Cotton swabs and mouthwashes are gentler ways to provide oral hygiene.

❑❑ **At what age do infants use up their prenatal iron stores from birth and require external sources?**

Age 4-6 months.

❑❑ **Iron drops are prescribed for a child. What food can be used to help aid in the absorption?**

Fruit juices. The vitamin C helps aid in absorption.

❑❑ **Why should medication not be mixed in a child's bottle as a method of administration?**

If the child does not finish the bottle, then you have no way of knowing how much of the medication was given.

❑❑ **What food should not be given with iron?**

Milk. It can decrease the absorption of Iron.

❑❑ **What foods contain a high amount of iron?**

Green vegetables, eggs, meats, and iron fortified cereals.

❑❑ **Why are children with iron deficiency anemia more prone to infection?**

The decreased iron decreases bone marrow functioning, and thus the production of white blood cells.

❑❑ **What is the most common cause of iron deficiency anemia in infants?**

Dietary deficiency. Usually the intake of milk is too high compared to the intake of solid foods. Milk does not contain enough iron to sustain the amount of iron needed.

❑❑ **How do you feed an infant who has just had surgical repair of a cleft palate?**
Any method that will cause the least amount of tension on their sutures. A medicine dropper is one example.

❑❑ **At what age is repair of the cleft palate done?**

Preferably before speech is able to develop.

❑❑ **How can you help the parents of a newborn with cleft palate accept the appearance of their child?**

Showing them pictures of the before and after results of surgery will give them a concrete picture of surgical expectations, support from other parents who have had children with cleft palate, encourage them to ask questions, and verbalize how they feel.

❑❑ **What is a priority nursing goal for an infant with a cleft palate?**

To provide adequate nutrition to the infant by finding alternative methods of feeding.

❑❑ **What is a common problem for a child following cleft palate surgery?**

Speech problems or deficit, often requiring speech therapy.

❑❑ **What is the best method for keeping the suture line free of debris following cleft palate surgery?**

A cotton swab moistened with saline or hydrogen peroxide.

❑❑ **What type of restraints are best for a child following some sort of surgery to the face?**

Elbow restraints. They restrict movement of the arms to the face, but are not too limiting to the child.

❑❑ **What abnormality found during pregnancy would alert the nurse to a possible gastrointestinal tract abnormality in the infant?**

Polyhydramnios.

❑❑ **What behavior would you expect a newborn to demonstrate when a transesophageal fistula (TEF) is present?**

The infant will attempt to feed normally, then will begin to cough, choke, and turn cyanotic as the contents swallowed are then returned through the nose and mouth.

❒❒ Because an infant with a cleft palate swallows large amounts of air when feeding, what should you do?

Burp the infant frequently when feeding him.

❒❒ Following surgery for cleft palate repair, the infant may have trouble breathing because he is not accustomed to nasal breathing. What should you do?

Exert pressure on the chin to open the mouth, or an artificial airway may need to be used.

❒❒ When irrigating a child's mouth following cleft palate surgery, what position should you place the child in?

Sitting up with the head foreword is the best way to prevent aspiration and choking.

❒❒ What physical clue would alert you that a child needs to be suctioned?

Accessory muscle breathing due to the laryngospasms caused by the build up of fluid in the lungs.

❒❒ How should you respond when parents of a child with a birth defect display guilt?

Encourage the parents to vent all their feelings and frustrations and answer their questions.

❒❒ When using a G-tube for feedings, how can you minimize air entering the stomach?

Keep the G-tube clamped until the feeding is ready to infuse, and re-clamp when the feeding finishes before air is introduced into the tube.

❒❒ What is a transesophageal fistula?

The upper esophagus ends in a blind pouch, and there is a fistula between the trachea and the lower esophagus.

❒❒ What physical symptoms would you see in a neonate with a transesophageal fistula?

Constant drooling and a lack of meconium stools due to the lack of ingestion of amniotic fluid while in utero.

❒❒ What position is best for an infant with TEF?

On their back with the upper body elevated. This reduces the flow of gastric juices into the lungs and allows for secretions to pool into the blind pouch.

❒❒ What long-term health problem should parents of a child with TEF be aware of?

The child may need corrective surgeries in the future for repair of an esophageal stricture that may develop at the anastomosis site.

❒❒ **What symptoms would alert you that an inguinal hernia is incarcerated?**

The hernia cannot be reduced, it is reddened, swollen, or painful.

❒❒ **What causes pyloric stenosis?**

Hypertrophy of the pylorus muscle distal to the stomach causing blockage of food contents trying to enter the stomach.

❒❒ **What does meconium passed in the urine indicate?**

A rectourinary fistula.

❒❒ **If an infant is not passing meconium stools, what is the possible cause?**

Imperforate anus or TEF.

❒❒ **What 3 electrolyte imbalances would you expect to see in a child who has been vomiting for a prolonged period of time?**

Hypokalemia, hyponatremia, and hypochloremia.

❒❒ **Will a child with an imperforate anus ever have normal bowel function?**

If the anomaly is located low in the intestinal tract, then chances are good that normal bowel function will be attained. With higher anomalies it is more difficult to attain normal sphincter control.

❒❒ **What acid-base imbalance should you watch for in a child who has been vomiting?**

Metabolic alkalosis.

❒❒ **Infants who are fed through a gastrostomy tube often lack what component of feeding?**

Physical closeness. You should hold them during the feeding.

❒❒ **How does a neonate respond to pain?**

Loud crying and total body movement rather than demonstrating localized pain in a certain area of the body.

❒❒ **What size of needle is best used for an infant receiving an injection?**

25-27 gauge, one-half inch to 1 inch in length.

❒❒ **After surgery for correction of an imperforate anus, how could you best keep tension off the perineum?**

Supine with the legs suspended, or lying on either side with the hips elevated.

❒❒ **The M.D. successfully reduces an infant's inguinal hernia and schedules surgery for 2 days later. Why is the surgery not performed immediately?**

To allow for reduction in swelling.

❒❒ You are assessing for Hirschsprung's disease. What should you look for?

History of abdominal distention, constipation, occasional diarrhea, and failure to thrive.

❒❒ What assessment findings could provide you with an infant's hydration status?

Intake and output, skin integrity, urine specific gravity, and daily weight.

❒❒ A child with severe dehydration is at risk for developing what acute kidney disorder?

Acute renal failure.

❒❒ What behavior would you expect to see in an infant with intussusception?

A shrill cry with the infant intermittently drawing the knees to the chest.

❒❒ For a child who is NPO with a nasogastric tube, how is IV fluid replacement determined?

Child's body weight and the amount of gastric contents lost.

❒❒ Why is surgical repair done to an inguinal hernia on an infant even if it is asymptomatic?

To prevent further complications that could be fatal to the child, such as an incarcerated bowel.

❒❒ How and where can you palpate a pyloric tumor?

In the epigastric region, just to the right of the umbilicus when the child's abdominal muscles are relaxed.

❒❒ Why are the stools of a child with intussusception often described as "currant jelly"?

The stools look like currant jelly due to the inflammation and hemorrhage associated with the intestinal obstruction.

❒❒ After abdominal surgery, a child develops an ileus. What would determine the return of bowel function?

Bowel sounds, passing of stool or gas, decrease in abdominal distention, and a decrease in the return of gastric contents from an NG tube.

❒❒ Following surgery for pyloric stenosis, when can an infant begin taking fluids?

Clear liquids may begin 6 hours post-op.

❒❒ What is the best position for an infant to promote gastric emptying?

On the right side with the head elevated.

❒❒ The vomitus of an infant with pyloric stenosis does not contain bile. Why?

The obstruction is proximal to the ampulla of vater where bile enters the stomach.

❑❑ **What is the most common post-op complication following inguinal hernia repair in an infant?**

Infection of the wound due to contamination by urine and stool.

❑❑ **Based on the above question, what should you teach the parents of a child prior to discharge after an inguinal hernia repair?**

Signs and symptoms of infection, and changing the diaper as soon as it becomes soiled.

❑❑ **How can you prepare a 6-month-old child for surgery emotionally and keep the child's anxiety level at a minimum?**

Have the primary caretaker stay with the child as much as possible to decrease the child's anxiety. However, there is no real way to prepare a child this young for the surgery.

❑❑ **What role does sucking provide for an infant?**

It is psychologically soothing, it provides comfort and security, and releases tension.

❑❑ **When can a child begin taking a bath following a surgery involving an external wound?**

About one week post op. Until then, a sponge bath should be given to avoid any chance of a wound infection developing.

❑❑ **An infant with Hirschsprung's disease undergoes a barium enema. How will you know if the barium is being expelled after the procedure?**

Clay colored stools indicate barium.

❑❑ **What is the primary defect of the intestinal tract in Hirschsprung's disease?**

There are no autonomic parasympathetic ganglion cells in the distal portion of the colon, therefore the normal motility of the intestinal tract is impaired.

❑❑ **Surgical repair of Hirschsprung's is accomplished by what method?**

Removal of the aganglionic bowel and the creation of a colostomy, which is usually reversed at 6-12 months of age after the bowel has rested and regained its original tone and size.

❑❑ **Following surgical repair for Hirschsprung's disease, you measure a child's abdomen for distention. What amount of distention in 8 hours would be cause for concern?**

3 cm or greater in 8 hours warrants physician notification.

❑❑ **Following abdominal surgery, a child is hungry, but bowel sounds cannot be heard. Should the child be fed anyway?**

No. Not until there is evidence of bowel function.

❑❑ **What type of diet is best for a child with a colostomy?**

A low residue diet.

❑❑ **What is the cause of cow's milk sensitivity in a newborn?**

It is an adverse local and systemic reaction to cow's milk protein. It usually resolves within 2 years of age.

❑❑ **What is phenylketonuria (PKU)?**

An autosomal recessive trait that prevents the conversion of phenylalanine to tyrosine. Any foods containing phenylalanine should be avoided.

❑❑ **What adverse affects occur if a child with PKU does not follow a restricted diet?**

Serum phenylalanine levels will elevate and this could lead to mental retardation.

❑❑ **Why is a newborn not tested for PKU until the first newborn check up in most cases?**

The infant must have ingested human or cow's milk for 4 days or more for the level of phenylalanine to be elevated.

❑❑ **At what age can a child with PKU begin a normal diet?**

It is not known. Some medical experts say the child should remain on this diet throughout life.

❑❑ **What foods should generally be limited in a child with PKU?**

Foods containing animal proteins.

❑❑ **What physical characteristics will you find in a child with PKU that will differ from other children?**

The skin color is light (due to the lower amounts of melanin), blue eyes, and light hair.

❑❑ **What are some of the clinical signs associated with an appendicitis?**

Right lower quadrant pain, localized tenderness, decreased or absent bowel sounds and fever.

❑❑ **What should be taken into consideration when assigning a room for a child with gastroenteritis?**

The child could be contagious and should be confined to a private room.

❑❑ **The M.D. orders that a child with diarrhea be made NPO even though the child is thirsty. Why?**

This allows for the gut to rest. Allowing the child to drink will only irritate the GI tract and prolong diarrhea. Fluids will be provided intravenously.

❑❑ **What does enteric precautions entail?**

A private room, gown when the nurse is in direct contact with the patient, and gloves when there is contact with stools.

❑❑ How is Salmonella typically spread?

Fecal-oral route from fowl, eggs, pet turtles, and kittens.

❑❑ When a child is dehydrated, you would expect the urine specific gravity to increase or decrease?

Increase.

❑❑ What are some of the symptoms of dehydration?

Dry mouth, decreased skin turgor, increased pulse, decreased tears and sweating, sunken eyes, decreased urine output and lethargy.

❑❑ Once a child with gastroenteritis is allowed to eat, what type of diet is usually instituted?

Clear liquids followed by the BRAT diet.

❑❑ What does the BRAT diet consist of and why does it work?

Bananas, rice, applesauce, and toast. These foods are easily digestible and are low in bulk, which helps in decreasing diarrhea.

❑❑ What should you say to a parent who is unable to stay with her child in the hospital because of other children at home?

Support the parent. Encourage involvement in the child's care by having her call or visit anytime. Do not make the parent feel guilty if there is no way he or she can stay with the child.

❑❑ You order a scalp IV for an infant. How should the parents be prepared before they see the child after IV insertion?

Explain that some hair will be shaved from the scalp and the reason for this. Parents are often upset with the physical appearance of their child. Reassure that the child is in no more discomfort than if the IV was in an extremity and the child's hair will grow back.

❑❑ You note that the IV site has become swollen and painful. What is the most likely reason?

The IV catheter has come out of the vein.

❑❑ What symptoms would lead you to suspect fluid overload from IV therapy?

Moist crackles heard upon auscultation of the lungs, dyspnea, increased blood pressure, intake greater that output, neck vein distention, cyanosis, and increased respiratory rate.

❑❑ What is the difference between lactose intolerance and milk sensitivity?

Lactose intolerance is caused by the lack of the enzyme lactase needed for digestion of lactose. Milk sensitivity is a local allergic reaction to milk that disappears as the child grows older.

❒❒ **What types of dairy products can the lactose intolerant child eat?**

Those that have been fermented such as yogurt, cheese, and buttermilk.

❒❒ **What is the accepted substitute for formula in milk sensitive children?**

Soy based formulas.

❒❒ **If a mother is breast-feeding, can her child still develop a milk sensitivity?**

Yes. The mother needs to be advised to eliminate all cow's milk from her diet.

❒❒ **A mother brings her child in and states, "He will eat anything on the floor, dirt, clay, and paint chips." What lab test would you want to check on this child?**

A lead blood test. Child with lead poisoning will often exhibit pica.

❒❒ **What complication could develop if lead poisoning goes untreated?**

Hematologic and renal effects can occur, but the most serious is mental retardation.

❒❒ **What is edetate disodium (EDTA) used for?**

Chelation therapy in lead poisoning.

❒❒ **What is syrup of ipecac?**

A medication used to induce vomiting.

❒❒ **How does syrup of ipecac work?**

It stimulates the vomiting center through direct irritation to the stomach mucosa.

❒❒ **Why are emetics contraindicated in the treatment for ingestion of caustic substances?**

The substance can cause further mucosa damage through vomiting.

❒❒ **What is a long-term complication following the ingestion of a caustic substance?**

Esophageal strictures caused by the formation of scar tissue.

❒❒ **A child has ingested a hydrocarbon such as kerosene. What complication should you be aware of?**

Respiratory complications resulting from a chemical pneumonitis caused by inhalation of the volatile hydrocarbon.

❒❒ **A patient brings in her infant with symptoms of colic. Why would you ask if there is anyone in the home who smokes?**

A higher incidence of colic has been reported in infants who live with a smoker.

❑❑ What are some techniques that may be helpful in calming an infant with colic?

Vibration, motion, smaller more frequent feedings, swaddling in a blanket, or a sedative.

❑❑ At what age does colic usually disappear?

3 months of age.

❑❑ What techniques could be taught that would help introduce less air into the intestines from feedings?

Feed the infant in an upright position, set in a car seat after feeding, and burp frequently during and after feeding.

❑❑ What is celiac disease?

An inherited intestinal disorder in which the infant is unable to digest glutan, part of the protein found in wheat, rye, barley, and oats.

❑❑ What would you expect the stools to look like in an infant with celiac disease?

Malodorous, pale, large, bulky, and loose.

❑❑ The parents of a child with celiac disease asks when their child will be able to eat normally. What is your response?

Never. This disease is not outgrown and the child will have to follow a restricted diet for the rest of his life.

❑❑ What physical finding would you expect to see in a patient with celiac disease?

A large, protruding abdomen.

❑❑ What is the physiological reason for the abdomen to protrude in a patient with celiac disease?

The intestines of the child are filled with gas and undigested food causing abdominal distension.

❑❑ Why should you be concerned with an adolescent who is obese?

Obesity in adolescence almost always leads to obesity into adulthood.

❑❑ What is the most accurate way to assess body fat?

Administering the skin-fold thickness test using skin calipers.

❑❑ An infant has been determined to be obese and is receiving an excessive amount of formula per day. How should the caloric intake be safely reduced?

Reduce the feeding to the recommended amount daily and use a smaller holed nipple.

❏❏ **At what age are solids generally introduced to infants?**

Age 4-6 months.

❏❏ **A client is concerned that her infant will eat more that he needs. How do you respond?**

An infant rarely eats more than he needs unless forced to do so. Watching for clues such as turning away or pushing out the nipple should be an indication that the infant is full.

❏❏ **What are some of the symptoms of a Urinary Tract Infection (UTI) in a young child?**

Irritability, fussiness, fever, abdominal pain, decreased appetite, dysuria, and increased frequency in urination.

❏❏ **A child is prescribed an antibiotic for treatment of a UTI and the parents ask how long her infant should take the medication. What is your response?**

Finish all the medication even if the symptoms disappear.

❏❏ **In a child, what method of urine collection results in the least amount of contamination?**

A suprapubic specimen.

❏❏ **A child with frequent UTIs is found to have vesicoureteral reflux. What is this?**

The vesicoureteral valve is incompetent and allows the reflux of urine from the bladder back into the ureter.

❏❏ **What special instruction should you give to the parents when their child is prescribed trimethoprim/sulfamethoxazole (Bactrim, Septra)?**

It causes photosensitivity, so the child should avoid prolonged exposure to the sun until the medication is finished.

❏❏ **Besides the white blood cell count, what results from a urinalysis would indicate a UTI?**

Protein, a pH greater than 8, leukocyte esterase, and nitrite.

❏❏ **What instructions can you give the parents to prevent the recurrence of a UTI?**

Increased fluid intake, wiping from front to back, avoiding bubble baths, voiding frequently, and wearing cotton underwear.

❏❏ **What is cryptorchidism?**

Failure of a testes to descend.

❏❏ **At what age do the testes usually descend?**

6 weeks.

❏❏ **What conditions are associated with an undescended testicle?**

Inguinal hernia, upper urinary tract anomalies, and a hydrocele, usually occurring on the same side as the affected testicle.

❑❑ **What is the cremasteric reflex?**

A reflex that causes the testicle to retract. Cold and touch can stimulate this.

❑❑ **What condition is more common in males who have had an undescended testicle as a child?**

Testicular cancer.

❑❑ **Knowing the above information, what should you include in your teaching plan for a male client with a history of an undescended testicle as a child?**

How to do a testicular self exam.

❑❑ **What is the purpose of applying traction to the testicles following surgery for cryptorchidism?**

To prevent the testicle from re-ascending.

❑❑ **What is nephrotic syndrome?**

It is an altered glomerular permeability that results in the excretion of large amounts of protein in the urine.

❑❑ **A child is allergic to penicillin and the physician orders amoxicillin. What should you do?**

Notify the physician of the penicillin allergy.

❑❑ **What is hypospadias?**

The urethral opening is located on the ventral surface of the penis or perineum.

❑❑ **How should an elastic bandage be wrapped around an extremity?**

Distal to proximal to facilitate venous drainage.

❑❑ **What is a Hydrocele?**

The collection of fluid in the tunica vaginalis of the testicle.

❑❑ **A child with a hydrocele is more susceptible to what lower abdominal condition?**

Inguinal hernia.

❑❑ **The parents of a child with hypospadias wish to have him circumcised. Why should you discourage this?**

The foreskin is often used to correct the deformity and thus circumcision should be avoided before corrective surgery.

❑❑ **What is enuresis?**

Bedwetting.

❑❑ **When a client has a restricted fluid intake, what is the best oral fluid to administer between meals?**

Ice chips.

❑❑ **What types of fluid increase thirst?**

Sweet beverages.

❑❑ **How is a hydrocele differentiated from an inguinal hernia?**

A hydrocele can be transiluminated. A hernia cannot because of the presence of intestines in the scrotal sac.

❑❑ **Following surgery for repair of a hydrocele, you order ice to be applied to the scrotum. Why?**

It decreases circulation to the area, thus preventing further swelling.

❑❑ **A client with glomerulonephritis has an elevated blood pressure. What should you be assessing for?**

Symptoms of hypertensive encephalopathy.

❑❑ **What are some of the symptoms of hypertensive encephalopathy?**

Elevated blood pressure, hemiparesis, loss of vision, disorientation, and seizures.

❑❑ **When the urinalysis is returned from a patient with glomerular nephritis, what results would you expect to see?**

Protein and RBC's in the urine.

❑❑ **A patient with glomerulonephritis is oliguric but has been placed on a fluid restriction. Why?**

In glomerulonephritis, the kidneys are no longer functioning normally and fluid that is taken in is retained. Edema, weight gain, and elevated blood pressure could result from the retention of fluids.

❑❑ **What is the most common type of glomerulonephritis in children?**

Post-streptococcal glomerulonephritis.

❑❑ **What is the preferred age to repair hypospadias?**

6-18 months of age or before the patient develops castration or body image anxiety.

❑❑ **A child returns from surgery after repair of hypospadias and his parents are upset that he has wrist restraints on. What should you do?**

Comfort the parents and explain the importance of the child not accidentally grabbing the catheters or stints involved in the surgical repair.

❑❑ **What types of catheters or stints should you prepare parents for that will be present after surgery for hypospadias?**

A urinary catheter or stint to maintain patency of the urethra, a suprapubic catheter for the drainage of urine, and an IV catheter for the infusion of fluids.

❑❑ **What is the most important comfort measure you can provide to an infant or young child who is immobile due to surgical restrictions?**

Having the parents stay at the bedside. Having the child see a familiar face close by will help reduce some of her/his anxiety.

❑❑ **What is the physiology of nephrotic syndrome?**

Altered glomerular permeability resulting in the excretion of a large amount of protein in the urine.

❑❑ **What is the most common cause of respiratory distress in nephrotic syndrome when no infection is present?**

Excess fluid in the abdominal cavity causes pressure on the diaphragm interfering with adequate chest expansion.

❑❑ **What type of diet is best for a child who has nephrotic syndrome?**

High protein and low sodium diet.

❑❑ **What is the most common type of intra-abdominal tumor of childhood?**

Wilm's tumor, or nephroblastoma.

❑❑ **What type of test is usually performed to determine the size and position of an abdominal tumor?**

Computerized tomography scan.

❑❑ **Following surgical removal of a Wilm's tumor, why should you teach the parents how to detect and prevent a urinary tract infection?**

The child has only one kidney so it should be protected from injury.

❑❑ **What are the advantages of peritoneal dialysis?**

There are no major diet restrictions, and it can be done at night when the patient is asleep.

❑❑ **What is the best sign indicating that fluid was left over after peritoneal dialysis?**

The patient's weight is higher after dialysis is completed.

❑❑ **When performing site care to the peritoneal catheter, what should you assess for?**

Signs and symptoms of infection at the exit site.

❒❒ What are the indications of an infection at the catheter exit site?

Redness, pain, swelling, and drainage.

❒❒ When peritonitis is present, what will the dialysate fluid look like?

Cloudy due to the large number of bacteria, fibrin, and white blood cells.

❒❒ What would be normal inflow and outflow drainage times for peritoneal dialysis?

10 minutes.

❒❒ Why should you not palpate a child's abdomen if Wilm's tumor is suspected?

It could cause dissemination of the tumor cells and thus spread the cancer.

❒❒ Following abdominal surgery, what intestinal problem could develop?

Intestinal obstruction due to an adynamic ileus.

❒❒ What symptoms should you look for when assessing for an intestinal obstruction?

Diminished or absent bowel sounds, vomiting, tachycardia, fever, shock, decreased urinary output, and hypotension.

❒❒ What medications are used to treat nephrotic syndrome?

Steroids, or cyclophosphamide.

❒❒ What are some of the side effects of cyclophosphamide?

Hair loss, nausea, decreased WBC count, cystitis, and possibly sterility.

❒❒ The parents are concerned because their child's eyelids have become so swollen from the edema associated with nephrotic syndrome. What could you suggest?

Elevating the head of the bed will help decrease some of the facial edema.

❒❒ Peritonitis is suspected in a child under going peritoneal dialysis. What lab test should you expect to be ordered on the dialysate fluid?

Culture and sensitivity.

❒❒ A child with edema often has pallor. What is the physiological cause of this?

Hemodilution.

❒❒ What other symptoms would you expect to find in a child with fluid overload?

Edema, elevated blood pressure, rales, and possible respiratory distress.

❑❑ **Why are intramuscular injections avoided in a child with a large amount of edema?**

The rate of absorption is slower.

❑❑ **What 2 methods, after surgical intervention, are the most common for treating Wilm's tumor?**

Chemotherapy and radiation.

❑❑ **How long after the initial treatment of chemotherapy does hair loss usually occur?**

2 weeks.

❑❑ **What position would be most comfortable for a child following abdominal surgery?**

Semi-fowlers.

❑❑ **You find an infant's head circumference to be in the 95th percentile, chest in the 60th percentile, and length in the 55th percentile. What should you asseses for next?**

Signs and symptoms of hydrocephalus.

❑❑ **What would you find if hydrocephalus were present?**

Bulging fontanels and widening cranial sutures.

❑❑ **What is the most common and the most dangerous complication following surgery for placement of a ventroperitoneal shunt?**

Infection.

❑❑ **If hydrocephalus is not corrected, what complication could result?**

Brain damage.

❑❑ **Following surgery for placement of a ventroperitoneal shunt, you place the infant supine at least for 24 hours. Why?**

Positioning the infant flat allows for the ventricles to drain slowly, allowing them to accommodate to the decreased fluid. If the drainage is too rapid it could cause a subdural hematoma.

❑❑ **What behavior in an infant would you expect if hydrocephalus is present?**

Lethargy, irritability, and difficulty in feeding due to a poor suck reflex.

❑❑ **An infant with a shunt in place begins to show signs of increased intercranial pressure. What would you suspect?**

A blocked shunt.

❑❑ **You compress the valve of the shunt, which compresses easily, but does not refill. Where is the**

blockage located?

The ventricular catheter is blocked.

❑❑ **Aminoglycoside antibiotics infused too rapidly can cause what side effect?**

Hypotension.

❑❑ **What is a meningocele?**

A soft sac containing only spinal fluid and meninges, located anywhere on the spine.

❑❑ **What is a myelomeningocele?**

Involves a bony defect, spinal fluid, and nerve tissue. It usually is found in the lower back, lying over the vertebrae with neurologic defects present.

❑❑ **What other cranial deformity is often associated with a myelomeningocele?**

Hydrocephalus.

❑❑ **The physician plans to repair the myelomeningocele defect immediately. How should you care for the defect site?**

Keep it moist with sterile saline gauze.

❑❑ **What would you expect in an infant with an upper myelomeningocele (L1-L2)?**

Dribbling of urine and feces, and minimal movement of the lower extremities.

❑❑ **What are the chances of a child with myelomeningocele being mentally retarded?**

One-third of the children with this disorder are mentally retarded.

❑❑ **Prior to closure, what is the nursing goal in caring for the spinal cord defect area?**

Protect it from pressure and potential infection.

❑❑ **What position is best in preventing injury to the spinal cord sac?**

A low Trendelenburg position with the hips slightly flexed, and the infant lying on his abdomen.

❑❑ **Since the dribbling of urine is common with myelomeningocele, how can you empty an infant's bladder in a way that has the lowest risk of infection?**

Apply gentle pressure above the suprapubic area and try to express the urine manually.

❑❑ **Children with a history of myelomeningocele are at risk for what types of infections?**

Urinary tract infections.

❑❑ **A child is admitted to the pediatric floor with suspected meningitis. Why is it important to get an accurate weight at this time?**

It will be used to calculate drug dosages.

❑❑ **What vital sign often increases along with increased intercranial pressure?**

The blood pressure.

❑❑ **Following a lumbar puncture in a small child, what should you do?**

Provide emotional support, preferably from someone the child trusts, apply a bandage to the site and hold pressure for a short period.

❑❑ **How long does a child need to lie flat following a lumbar puncture?**

The child does not need to lie flat. It is not necessary and probably impossible.

❑❑ **How does a child usually contract bacterial meningitis?**

Spread by vascular dissemination from a middle ear or sinus infection.

❑❑ **What behavior would you expect in a child with meningitis?**

Irritability, and hypersensitivity to light and noise.

❑❑ **What simple nursing measure can be done if you suspect increasing intercranial pressure?**

Elevate the head of the bed. Neck flexion or extension should be avoided because it can inhibit venous return.

❑❑ **Disseminated intravascular coagulation (DIC) is a potential complication of meningitis. What is the early sign of this disorder?**

Hemorrhagic skin rash.

❑❑ **A child with a severe head injury is brought into the ED. What is your first priority in assessment?**

Establish the patency of the airway. Remember the ABC's

❑❑ **Why is a nasogastric tube inserted when a client has severe head trauma?**

To decompress the stomach and prevent aspiration. The risk of aspiration is greater in an unconscious client.

❑❑ **In what type of fracture would an oral, rather than nasogastric, tube be recommended?**

A basilar skull fracture. Inserting the tube nasally could be dangerous since the tube could accidentally be inserted through the fracture into the soft tissue.

❑❑ **What is the purpose of mannitol in treating head trauma?**

It is an osmotic diuretic used to decrease intracranial pressure caused by cerebral edema.

❑❑ **A child has been found to have a mild concussion and is sent home. For what symptoms should you instruct the parents to watch out?**

Vomiting 3 or more times, abnormal behavior, excruciating headache that interferes with sleep, or an inability to arouse from sleep.

❑❑ **Should a child be allowed to sleep after being diagnosed with possible concussion?**

Yes. There is no contraindication to sleep.

❑❑ **When does spinal shock usually occur?**

30 to 60 minutes following a spinal cord injury due to interruption of central and autonomic pathways.

❑❑ **What are some of the symptoms of spinal shock?**

Loss of reflexes below the level of injury, vasodilatation, hypotension, increased pulse and respirations, and flaccid paralysis.

❑❑ **What is expected to be the common response of a patient following a catastrophic injury?**

Denial, anger, shock, and depression.

❑❑ **During the acute phase of a spinal cord injury, why should you assess the patient's abdomen?**

To observe for signs of a paralytic ileus.

❑❑ **What will you most likely observe when spinal shock begins to resolve?**

The return of reflexes, however, they are usually hyperactive.

❑❑ **What is your priority when a client is having a seizure?**

Protect the patient from injury, and maintain an open airway.

❑❑ **What is the most common cause of status epilepticus?**

Withdrawal of anticonvulsant medication.

❑❑ **Following a seizure, a child is difficult to arouse and is incontinent of urine. What is this period called?**

Post-ictal.

❑❑ **Should you attempt to arouse a patient during the post-ictal stage?**

Client's are often difficult to arouse during this period and it is OK to allow them to sleep.

❑❑ **What special precautions regarding phenytoin sodium (Dilantin) and over the counter drugs should be included in nurse teaching?**

Phenytoin sodium (Dilantin) interacts with many over the counter medications so they should never be taken without consulting a physician first.

❑❑ **While taking phenytoin sodium (Dilantin), the parent notes a pink tinge to the child's urine. What should you do?**

Tell the patient this is a normal side effect of the drug.

❑❑ **What teaching should you do in regards to administration of anticonvulsant medications?**

Always take the prescribed dose. Medication should never be made up for, discontinued, or missed as this could alter the therapeutic blood level.

❑❑ **What is the best teaching advice to give parents in regards to helping their child through a seizure?**

Stay with the child and help prevent any injury from occurring. Restraining the child or forcing objects into her mouth will only cause injury.

❑❑ **The parent's of a child with a seizure disorder are concerned about her ability to attend a public school. How should you respond?**

There is no reason why the child cannot attend a regular school. Intellectually, the child will be normal and she needs the same experiences as other children.

❑❑ **Liquid anti-seizure medication is usually avoided in children for what reason?**

The accuracy in dosage is decreased.

❑❑ **What side effect can occur from rapidly infusing phenytoin sodium (Dilantin)?**

Cardiotoxicity leading to bradycardia, hypotension, cardiac arrest, and asystole.

❑❑ **What methods should be avoided when trying to lower body temperature?**

Alcohol sponge baths and placing the child into cold bath water. Both methods will only serve to increase body temperature, and the alcohol can be toxic.

❑❑ **Does a child with febrile seizures need long-term anticonvulsant medication?**

No.

❑❑ **When do febrile seizures usually occur?**

During a rapid temperature rise that usually involves the presence of some sort of upper respiratory infection. Febrile seizures are also familial.

❑❑ **What is the cause of Reye's syndrome?**

The cause if unknown. But it is known that it develops after a viral illness, the administration of salicylates can contribute to its development, and it is not communicable.

❑❑ **In a child with Reye's syndrome, what nursing measures can be taken to decrease the child's agitation?**

Avoid all loud or unnecessary stimuli.

❑❑ **If a child with Reye's syndrome continues to deteriorate, what symptom should you prepare for?**

The onset of seizures.

❑❑ **A child is admitted with possible Guillain-Barre Syndrome. Why would you want to assess muscle strength?**

Determine which muscles are involved and if the disorder progressing.

❑❑ **What is another name for Guillain-Barre Syndrome?**

Infectious polyneuritis.

❑❑ **Is it possible to recover from Guillain-Barre?**

Yes, but the rehabilitation is lengthy. It is usually 1-2 years for a full recovery.

❑❑ **Why should a child with Guillain-Barre be handled gently when nursing care is given?**

The child may be immobile because of the effects of this disease, but he can still feel. In fact, hypersensitivity to touch is often common.

❑❑ **You test a Guillain-Barre child's gag and cough reflex. What are you assessing for?**

Cranial nerve involvement.

❑❑ **When Guillain-Barre syndrome affects a child's autonomic nervous system, why is it important for the child to be placed on a cardiac monitor?**

There is the potential for cardiac dysrhythmias to occur.

❑❑ **A child is placed on NG tube feedings after losing his gag reflex. How can you determine when he can resume oral feedings?**

Assess for the return of the gag reflex by gently inserting an object, such as a tongue depressor, in the back of his throat.

❑❑ **What should you suspect in a child with the following symptoms: headache, visual disturbances, vomiting, neurological deficits, and ataxia?**

Possible brain tumor.

❑❑ **How can you help the parents of a child with a brain tumor cope with their fears?**

Giving information about the disease, explaining all procedures, and offering emotional support.

❑❑ What does the term "Stage I" indicate when referring to a brain tumor?

The tumor is localized and there is no evidence of spread. This is the lowest stage and has the best prognosis.

❑❑ Following removal of an infratentorial brain tumor, what is the best position for a child to be placed?

Flat, with the neck in line with the body to decrease intercranial pressure.

❑❑ Why would the Trendelenburg position be contraindicated after brain tumor removal?

This could cause an increase in intercranial pressure.

❑❑ Following head trauma, the physician orders an intubated child to be hyperventilated. What is the purpose of this?

A decreased pCO_2 and increased pO_2 will decrease intercranial pressure.

❑❑ Following a craniotomy, you note clear fluid drainage on the dressings. What should you test this fluid for?

Glucose. This would indicate the presence of CSF fluid.

❑❑ How is Duchenne's muscular dystrophy contracted?

It is an x-linked genetic disorder.

❑❑ While assessing a child with muscular dystrophy, you note Gower's sign. What is this?

Walking the hands up the legs in an attempt to stand from a sitting position.

❑❑ What is the most common musculo-skeletal problem that occurs as a result of muscular dystrophy?

Skeletal contractures resulting from the lack of movement of certain joints due to selective muscle involvement.

❑❑ What is the most common cause of death in children with muscular dystrophy?

Death from cardiac disease or respiratory tract infection.

❑❑ What are the early clinical signs of a child with muscular dystrophy?

Difficulty climbing stairs, running, or riding a bike.

❑❑ The mother of a child with muscular dystrophy asks how she can prevent her child from getting worse. How should you respond?

Muscular dystrophy is progressive. The longer the child is active, the longer it may prolong wheelchair use, but inevitably the child will end up wheelchair bound.

❑❑ **Knowing the trait for muscular dystrophy is usually passed from mother to son, what possible feelings should you be aware of in the patient's mother?**

Feelings of guilt which are common in any genetic disorder. The parent often feels responsible for bringing this upon the child.

❑❑ **What are the signs and symptoms of osteomyelitis?**

Localized tenderness, increased warmth, swelling over the affected bone, and redness.

❑❑ **What is the usual treatment for osteomyelitis?**

3-4 weeks of IV antibiotics.

❑❑ **Before antibiotic therapy is started, what test would the physician order to help determine the causative organism?**

Blood cultures.

❑❑ **What lab values would you expect to be elevated in a child with osteomyelitis?**

WBC count and sedimentation rate.

❑❑ **What does the presence of an elevated sedimentation rate indicate?**

The presence of a localized or systemic infection.

❑❑ **What body systems can be affected by long-term antibiotic therapy?**

Renal and hepatic.

❑❑ **What is the most effective method of preventing skin breakdown in a child confined to bed?**

Frequently changing position.

❑❑ **If a child has osteomyelitis in the lower tibia, how should you position the affected limb?**

Elevated with warm moist packs to the affected area to help decrease swelling.

❑❑ **What is Legg-Calve-Perthes disease?**

Osteochondrosis, or aseptic necrosis of the head of the femur.

❑❑ **What would you expect to find if a child has kyphosis of the spine?**

An abnormal curvature of spine, usually convex in nature.

❑❑ **What is torticollis?**

Limited range of motion in the neck characterized by the head being turned to one side and the chin pointing to the other side.

❑❑ **Which muscle is involved in torticollis?**

The sternocleidomastoid muscle.

❑❑ **A child is diagnosed with Osgood-Schlatter disease. What other term is used to describe this disease?**

Growing pains.

❑❑ **What part of the body does Osgood-Schlatter's disease occur?**

The tibial tuberosity.

❑❑ **What would you look for when assessing for scoliosis?**

With the child bending forward at the waist, a lateral curvature of the thoracic spine would be present along with a rib hump.

❑❑ **What is the usual treatment for scoliosis?**

The Milwaukee brace.

❑❑ **How often can a child remove a Milwaukee brace?**

The brace must be worn at all times and can only be removed for bathing.

❑❑ **What is the goal of treatment for a child with Legg-Calve-Perthes disease?**

Keep pressure off the head of the femur, which would cause more damage.

❑❑ **What is the treatment for flat feet?**

Generally there is no treatment, although corrective shoes are sometimes prescribed.

❑❑ **What should you assess for after application of a cast?**

Determine vascular compromise by assessing color, temperature, sensation, and capillary refill of the extremity distal to the cast.

❑❑ **What is the usual treatment for a club foot deformity?**

A series of plaster casts that will move the foot into a normal position. Sometimes, surgery is indicated in severe cases.

❑❑ **When handling a newly applied cast, you are careful not to handle the cast with your fingertips. Why?**

This could leave indentations in the cast which could put pressure on the soft tissue underneath. Handle with your palms only.

❑❑ **Why is it not advised to dry a cast with the use of a blow dryer?**

This dries the surface of the cast only, leaving the inside damp. It could also lead to the transfer of heat through the cast and cause burns to the skin.

❑❑ **If you suspect child abuse, but you are not sure, should it be reported?**

Yes. It is your legal obligation.

❑❑ **Following a fall, a 2-year-old child is brought to the ED with a swollen, bruised wrist. A possible fracture is suspected. What should you assess in relation to this?**

Assess the area distal to the possible fracture for sign of neurovascular compromise.

❑❑ **What is the purpose of traction in treating a fracture?**

Its purpose is to align and immobilize bone fragments, which will help prevent further tissue injury and relieve muscle spasms.

❑❑ **When a fracture occurs, what is the normal response of the surrounding muscles?**

To contract. It is the body's natural response to try to immobilize the fracture.

❑❑ **A 5-year-old child with a fracture is apprehensive and uncooperative when the physician attempts to cast his arm. What can you do to help alleviate fears?**

Give the child instructions as to what is going to be done in language he can understand. Have the parents stay for emotional support.

❑❑ **After casting, what discharge instructions should you give the parents?**

Signs and symptoms of vascular compromise, cast care instructions, and how to care for the cast until it fully dries.

❑❑ **Until the cast is fully dry, what type of material should the cast extremity lie on when the child is resting?**

A soft surface, such as pillows, that will not dent or flatten the cast.

❑❑ **What does a positive Ortolani's sign indicate in an infant?**

Congenital hip dislocation. It is the feeling of the femoral head slipping forward into the acetabulum when pressure is exerted from behind the greater trochanter and the knee is held laterally.

❑❑ **With hip dysplasia, there is also a shortening of the limb on the affected side. This is known as what sign?**

Galleazzi's sign.

❑❑ **If a congenital hip is to be treated by casting, what type of cast is usually applied?**

A spica cast.

❑❑ **You teach the parents to apply pieces of overlapping tape to the edges of the cast. What is the purpose of this?**

Prevent skin irritation from the rough cast edges.

❑❑ **Is there a contraindication to breast feeding in a child with a spica cast?**

No, although alternate positions for breastfeeding may have to be taught to the mother.

❑❑ **Three weeks after applying the spica cast, you note that the child's toes are cool and swollen. If there is no sign of infection, what should you suspect is the cause?**

The child has outgrown the cast. Infants grow rapidly and casts frequently have to be changed.

❑❑ **What is the term that describes a collective range of neuromuscular problems related to tone and/or function, that are non-progressive and are the result of cerebellar damage?**

Cerebral palsy.

❑❑ **What term would describe a child that had paralysis on one side of the body?**

Hemiparesis.

❑❑ **You note increased muscle tone in the calf and right forearm, and persistent reflexes in an infant with a history of cerebral anoxia. What type of cerebral palsy would this be?**

Spastic cerebral palsy.

❑❑ **When initial screening is done on a child with cerebral palsy, why is it so important for you to identify the primary developmental delays?**

Recognizing the primary developmental delays will help plan care that will prevent secondary and tertiary developmental delays.

❑❑ **What term is used to describe paralysis of all 4 extremities?**

Quadriplegia.

❑❑ **You offer toys to a child with hemiplegia to his affected side. What is the purpose in doing this?**

To encourage the child to use his affected limb.

❑❑ **What lab test is used to diagnose juvenile rheumatoid arthritis (JRA)?**

There is no definitive test.

❑❑ **What is the prognosis of JRA?**

Most children are in complete remission by adolescence, some may go into remission before that time, but rarely will the child see recovery within the first few years of the disease.

❑❑ How can parents help their child with JRA increase his mobility in the affected joints?

Specific exercises and the application of heat to affected joints is used to increase mobility.

❑❑ What type of traction is Bryant's traction - skin or skeletal?

Skin.

❑❑ A child with a femur fracture is placed in Bryant's traction and you wish to change the dressing at the traction site. Should the weights to the traction be removed to accomplish this task?

You should never remove or add weights or change the moleskin used for the skeletal traction unless specifically ordered to do so.

❑❑ What assessment should you do on a child in traction?

Cardiovascular status of the affected extremity.

❑❑ A mother states she has been applying lotion under the edges of her child's cast. What should you instruct her to do?

Don't apply lotion because it causes skin irritation and breakdown because of the increased moisture.

❑❑ The parent of a toddler with an arm cast calls and states that the child went swimming with the cast on. What should you advise the parent?

Come in for a cast change.

❑❑ A child with a fractured femur suddenly complains of chest pain, is diaphoretic, tachycardic, and dyspneic. What should you suspect?

Pulmonary embolus most likely from a fat embolus from the fracture site.

❑❑ A child with a spica cast complains it is too tight after eating a meal. What could you suggest?

Eat smaller, more frequent meals to decrease abdominal distention.

❑❑ In the immediate post-casting period, what is the highest nursing priority in patient assessment?

Assessing for signs and symptoms of neurovascular compromise to the affected extremity.

❑❑ What are the 3 cardinal signs of diabetes?

Polydipsia, polyuria, and polyphagia.

❑❑ What is the characteristic breathing pattern of someone in ketoacidosis?

Kussmaul's breathing.

❑❑ **What is the physiological reasoning behind Kussmaul's breathing?**

Ketones cause the patient's blood to become acidotic (blood pH is low). The body attempts to compensate by ridding itself of any excess acid (H+ ions). By getting rid of excess carbon dioxide, more acid is blown off and the blood pH will begin to rise.

❑❑ **The parents of a child with Diabetes Mellitus (DM) ask, "Why can't my child just take a pill of insulin rather than injecting it?" How should you respond?**

Insulin is destroyed by digestive enzymes. There are oral hypoglycemics, but they are not effective in clients with DM.

❑❑ **What causes the characteristic breath odor in a child with diabetic ketoacidosis?**

The release of acetone caused by the breakdown of fats during fat metabolism and the build-up of ketones, a by-product of that metabolism.

❑❑ **When mixing insulin for an insulin drip, what IV solution should be used?**

Normal (0.9%) saline.

❑❑ **The physician orders 100 units of NPH insulin in 100 cc of normal saline. Why would you question this order?**

Only regular insulin is given intravenously.

❑❑ **You instruct a 13-year-old with insulin-dependent diabetes mellitus (IDDM) not to inject his insulin into his thighs before track practice. Why?**

Increased blood supply to the surrounding tissues from exercise could cause the insulin to be absorbed quicker than usual.

❑❑ **What should the parents of a child with IDDM be instructed in?**

The signs and symptoms of hypoglycemia and the appropriate actions to take.

❑❑ **Before connecting an IV solution containing insulin and normal saline to a patient, you make sure the IV tubing has been completely flushed with the insulin/normal saline solution. Why?**

Insulin sticks to the plastic tubing. Flushing it first ensures that solution containing insulin is being administered to the patient as soon as the infusion is started.

❑❑ **Why is it important for a patient with (IDDM) to be taught to rotate the site of injection?**

Using the same site over and over can result in fat atrophy and thus lead to poor absorption of insulin.

❑❑ **When would you expect to see the results of lente insulin after injection?**

2-4 hours after injection and peaks at 6-8 hours.

❑❑ **Why is it important to include snacks in the diabetic diet?**

Snacks are usually given at times that will offset the periods of peak insulin action.

❑❑ **The nurse determines a child is having a hypoglycemic reaction. What should be done?**

Administer some form of simple sugar immediately.

❑❑ **What is the basic principle behind the diabetic exchange diet?**

That certain foods have similar fat, protein, and carbohydrate components and can be substituted freely as long as the patient stays within the allotted number of allowed exchanges from each category.

❑❑ **What is lanugo?**

Fine hair that covers the entire body of the infant until about 20 weeks gestation. From then on it begins to deteriorate.

❑❑ **Why is it important that you keep a record of the amount of blood drawn from a preterm infant?**

The blood volume in preterm infants is limited and too many blood collections can lead to blood volume depletion.

❑❑ **Preterm infants are often at risk for developing what metabolic condition?**

Cold stress.

❑❑ **In cold stress, you would be alert to signs of hyperactivity or muscle twitching which could indicate what condition?**

Hypoglycemia.

❑❑ **Why do preterm infants often develop cold stress?**

The infant is trying to produce enough heat to keep warm, but its glycogen stores are used up quickly, thus hypoglycemia and metabolic acidosis can result.

❑❑ **Why would sodium bicarbonate be given to an infant with cold stress?**

To eliminate metabolic acidosis.

❑❑ **What is the complication associated with a high level of oxygen administration in neonates?**

Retrolental fibroplasia.

❑❑ **How can you determine if a gavage-feeding catheter is in the correct position?**

Aspiration of stomach contents or auscultation of air introduced into the stomach via the catheter.

❑❑ **Why is it important to return stomach contents to the stomach after aspirating?**

Loss of fluids and electrolytes can be significant, especially in the neonate, if the contents are not returned.

❑❑ **What is the single most useful technique in preventing the spread of infection on a pediatric unit?**

Handwashing.

❑❑ **What is the determining factor in diagnosing failure to thrive?**

Comparing an infant's growth weight with those of the same age. Generally, if the infant falls below the 5th percentile, it is considered "failure to thrive."

❑❑ **How would you expect an infant with the diagnosis of failure to thrive to behave during feedings?**

The infant will usually be fussy during feedings and sometimes be difficult to feed.

❑❑ **One of the nursing goals for a failure to thrive infant is to develop positive feeding patterns. How is this best accomplished?**

Have the same nurse feed the infant as much as possible. The parents should not feed the infant until it has gained an acceptable amount of weight. Holding and cuddling the infant before and after the feeding are helpful.

❑❑ **When calculating the percent of body surface burned in a child, how should you alter your calculations from an adult?**

Since the head is much larger in the child, the head is equal to 9% plus 1% for each year under 12. Each lower extremity is 18% in an adult, but in the child, subtract 0.5% for each year under 12.

❑❑ **Following a severe burn, what type of diet should a child be placed on?**

A diet high in protein, calories, and iron.

❑❑ **You prepare to administer a large amount of IV fluids to a burn victim because you understand that there will be a large fluid shift from what physiological space?**

From the intravascular to the interstitial spaces.

❑❑ **What is the importance of having an indwelling catheter in a burn victim?**

Urine output is used as an indicator of fluid volume status and in calculating fluid replacement therapy.

❑❑ **Along with urine output, you can also perform what other test on a patient's urine to determine fluid status?**

Urine specific gravity.

❑❑ **You assess a burn client's lungs and hear moist rales. What could this indicate if the patient is still receiving IV therapy?**

Fluid overload is occurring.

❑❑ **A 6-year-old child becomes combative and uncooperative when it is time to change his burn**

dressings. You allow him to help with the dressing change, and he calms down. Why?

The child's behavior was probably a result of a feeling of a loss of control. Allowing the child to assist with dressing changes gave him back some of that control.

❑❑ You are administering an IV antibiotic, when you note redness and raised welts accompanied by itching on the patient's arm. What should you do?

Stop the infusion and notify the M.D. The patient could be having an allergic reaction.

❑❑ Which juice is helpful in elevating serum potassium?

Orange juice.

❑❑ A 2-year-old child is brought to the ED with a broken leg. Throughout the exam and during the blood draw, the child lies still and does not complain. What should you suspect?

The possibility of child abuse, especially if the fracture is suspicious and there is no medical reason for why the child is so passive to pain.

❑❑ When suspecting child abuse, what are some important assessments that should be documented on the patient's chart?

The behavior of the patient and any physical findings. These will be important if the case goes to court.

❑❑ If a child confides to you that he or she has been abused, but the abuse is denied by the parents, what should you do?

The child must be believed and the case will have to be reported.

❑❑ A fellow nurse states that she suspects child abuse with one of her clients, but fears reporting it because the patient's father is a lawyer. How should you respond to this nurse?

A health care professional cannot be sued for reporting a suspected child abuse case.

❑❑ What are the most common foods that infants can be allergic to?

Eggs and cow's milk.

❑❑ A 2-year-old child has puritic eczema and you choose long sleeve cotton pajamas for the child to wear at night. What is the reasoning behind this?

Long sleeves will prevent the child from scratching his extremities, and cotton is preferred over other materials for puritis.

❑❑ An infant is brought to the ED with a high fever and lethargy. You become concerned when the infant's heart rate increases to 210 and his temperature begins to fall. Why?

These signs could indicate septic shock.

❑❑ Why is a diaphragmatic hernia in a neonate considered a surgical emergency?

Abdominal contents may compress and displace the lungs and heart leading to respiratory distress.

❑❑ **What are the indications that a mother's milk supply is adequate for a breast-fed infant?**

The child will appear content, have good skin turgor, an adequate number of wet diapers, and normal weight gain.

❑❑ **Strawberry hemangiomas are raised red birthmarks that may continue to spread up to age one. Complete shrinkage and absorption may take up to how long?**

7-10 years.

❑❑ **What is the Guthrie test?**

A screening test for PKU.

❑❑ **When is the Guthrie test most sensitive?**

It is most reliable if it is done between the second and sixth day after birth and after the neonate has ingested protein.

❑❑ **How do you assess the rooting reflex?**

You touch a finger to the neonate's cheek or corner of its mouth. Normally, the neonate will turn his head towards the stimulus, open the mouth, and search for the stimulus.

❑❑ **What is the leading cause of poisoning in children?**

Aspirin ingestion.

❑❑ **Why should cow's milk not be given in the first year of life?**

The protein is difficult for infants to digest and it has a low linoleic acid content.

❑❑ **What is the first sign of respiratory distress in a premature infant?**

Nasal flaring.

❑❑ **What is the first sign of lead poisoning in a child?**

Anemia.

❑❑ **What is the most common cancer during childhood?**

Leukemia.

❑❑ **What is one of the most common causes of child abuse?**

Poor impulse control by the parent.

❑❑ **What is the most appropriate toy for a toddler age 18 months?**

A toy that helps to develop motor coordination.

❒❒ **What position should an infant be placed in after breast-feeding?**

On their side.

❒❒ **What is the most common brain tumor in a child?**

Medulloblastoma.

❒❒ **What is Von Willebrand's disease?**

It is an autosomal-dominant bleeding disorder that results from platelet dysfunction and Factor VIII deficiency.

❒❒ **What is the definition of a premature infant?**

An infant born before the end of the 37th week of gestation.

❒❒ **What is the definition of a low-birth-weight infant?**

1,500-2,500 grams (3 pounds, 5 ounces to 5 pounds, 8 ounces) at birth regardless of gestational age.

❒❒ **What is the leading cause of death among teenagers?**

Suicide.

❒❒ **At what age do infants double their birth weight?**

Most double their birth weight by age 5 to 6 months and triple it by age 1.

❒❒ **What is the most common chromosomal disorder?**

Down's syndrome (trisomy 21).

❒❒ **What are the signs and symptoms of pyloric stenosis?**

Palpable olive-sized mass in the right upper quadrant, strong peristaltic movements from the left to right, and projectile vomiting.

❒❒ **After feeding an infant with a cleft lip or palate, you should do what?**

Rinse the infant's mouth with sterile water.

❒❒ **What infection is an infant with a cleft palate at risk of developing?**

Otitis media.

❒❒ **Why is toilet training unsuccessful during the first 2 years of life?**

The infant has minimal sphincter control until around age 2.

❑❑ **What are the first signs of respiratory distress in a toddler?**

Increased respiratory rate and pulse.

❑❑ **What position should a child with ascites from chronic liver disease be placed in to promote respiratory functioning?**

Semi-Fowler's.

❑❑ **What type of a cry is heard from infants with hydrocephalus?**

High-pitched shrill.

❑❑ **What is the leading cause of death in children?**

Accidents.

❑❑ **According to Freud, when does the oral stage occur?**

Birth to age 18 months.

❑❑ **What is the most serious and irreversible consequence of lead poisoning?**

Mental retardation.

❑❑ **Teratology of Fallot consists of what 4 defects.**

Ventricular septal defect, overriding aorta, pulmonic stenosis, and right ventricular hypertrophy.

❑❑ **According to Erikson, the identity-versus-role confusion state occurs when?**

Ages 12 and 20.

❑❑ **How do you prevent urine from running under a Spica cast?**

Elevate the head of the patient's bed higher than the foot of the bed.

❑❑ **What are the typical findings seen in an infant with Down's syndrome?**

Hypotonia, foppiness, slanted eyes, excess skin on the back of the neck, flattened bridge of the nose, flat facial features, short and broad feet, spade-like hands, small genitalia, and simian palmar creases.

❑❑ **What period is considered the infancy period?**

Birth to 1 year of age.

❑❑ **What age is the toddler stage?**

Age 1-3.

❑❑ **When should breast feeding begin?**

As soon as possible after delivery.

❑❑ **What is the most common disorder of the hip joint in a patient under 3 years of age?**

Congenital hip dysplasia.

❑❑ **What type of diet should be prescribed for a patient with celiac disease?**

Gluten-free diet.

❑❑ **When taking a child's temperature rectally, how far should you insert the thermometer?**

One-half inch.

❑❑ **Most infants born with HIV positive blood develop AIDS when?**

2-4 months.

❑❑ **What diagnostic test is used to confirm the diagnosis of cystic fibrosis?**

Sweat test.

❑❑ **What is the drug of choice for treating attention deficit disorder in hyperactive children?**

Methylphenidate hydrochloride (Ritalin).

❑❑ **What parts of the infant body should be covered during phototherapy?**

The infant's eyes and genital area.

❑❑ **How often should a child have a fluoride treatment?**

Twice a year.

❑❑ **What are the symptoms of respiratory distress syndrome in a neonate?**

Expiratory grunting, harsh breath sounds, and retractions.

❑❑ **What are the signs and symptoms of acute rheumatic fever?**

Chorea, fever, carditis, migratory polyarthritides, erythema marginatum, and subcutaneous nodules.

❑❑ **What are the most common disorders of infants born to diabetic women?**

Skeletal system abnormalities and ventricular septal defects.

❑❑ **What is phimosis?**

Tightening of the prepuce of the penis that prevents foreskin retraction over the glans.

❑❑ **After surgical reconstruction of an imperforate anus, an infant should be placed in what position?**

Prone with the hips elevated.

❒❒ **At what age does object permanence develop?**

6-8 months.

❒❒ **What does "molding" refer to during the birth process?**

The process by which the fetal head changes shape to facilitate movement through the birth canal.

❒❒ **What is the most common fracture in children?**

Greenstick fracture.

❒❒ **What patient care measures should be taken during a sickle cell crisis?**

Bedrest, IV fluids, oxygen, analgesics, and a thorough documentation of fluid intake and output.

❒❒ **An infant presents for her immunizations but has a fever. What should be done?**

Immunization should be postponed.

❒❒ **According to Erikson, at what age does the developmental age of integrity versus despair occur?**

Age 65 or older.

❒❒ **What is impetigo?**

A contagious, superficial vesiculopustular skin infection.

❒❒ **A neonate is born with meconium ileus resulting in an obstruction of the small intestine. What disorder must be considered?**

Cystic fibrosis.

❒❒ **What is the initial weight loss for a healthy neonate?**

5-10% of the birth weight.

❒❒ **What is the most common intra-abdominal tumor in children?**

Wilms' tumor.

❒❒ **What are the early signs of a congenital heart defect in an infant?**

Fatigue, tachypnea, irritability during feeding, and other assorted feeding problems.

❒❒ **Bath water should not exceed what temperature?**

105 degrees Fahrenheit (40.5 degrees Celsius).

MENTAL HEALTH PEARLS

"Examinations are formidable event to the best prepared,
for the greatest fool may ask more than the wisest man can answer."
Unknown

❑❑ **What is the typical profile of a patient with anorexia nervosa?**

Female, adolescent, upper class, and perfectionist.

❑❑ **A patient with an eating disorder often unconsciously associates food with what emotion?**

Love and affection.

❑❑ **Differentiate between Korsakoff's psychosis and Wernicke's encephalopathy.**

Korsakoff's psychosis: Inability to process new information (i.e., to form new memories). This is a reversible condition resulting from brain damage induced by a thiamine deficiency which is generally secondary to chronic alcoholism.

Wernicke's encephalopathy: This disease is also due to an alcoholic-induced thiamine deficiency. It is an irreversible disease in which the brain tissues break down, become inflamed, and bleed. Patients have decreased muscle coordination, ophthalmoplegia, and confusion.

❑❑ **A 32-year-old female is given meperidine (Demerol) for an open fracture. The patient is chronically on fluoxetine (Prozac). What is a potential complication?**

The serotonin syndrome.

❑❑ **What signs and symptoms are typical of the serotonin syndrome?**

Agitation, anxiety, sinus tachycardia, shivering, tremor, hyperreflexia, myoclonus, muscular rigidity, and diarrhea.

❑❑ **What lithium level is generally considered toxic?**

2.0 mEq/L.

❑❑ **What are the signs and symptoms of lithium toxicity?**

Neurological signs and symptoms include tremor, hyperreflexia, clonus, fasciculations, seizures, and coma. GI signs and symptoms consist of nausea, vomiting, and diarrhea. Finally, signs and symptoms associated with CV are ST-T wave changes, bradycardia, conduction defects, and arrhythmias.

❑❑ **What is the pharmacological treatment of alcohol withdrawal?**

Benzodiazepines or barbiturates.

❒❒ **What is the Sundown Syndrome in the elderly?**

Hallucinations and delusions that occur at night.

❒❒ **What is the most common nontraumatic cause of dementia?**

Alzheimer's disease. At 65, 10% of the population has Alzheimer's; by 85, the percentage increases to 50%. Multi-infarct dementia is the second most common cause of nontraumatic dementia.

❒❒ **What is the first symptom of Alzheimer's disease?**

Progressive memory loss. This is followed by disorientation, personality changes, language difficulty, and other symptoms of dementia.

❒❒ **What is the prognosis for patients with Alzheimer's disease?**

This is an irreversible disease. Death occurs 5–10 years after presumptive diagnosis.

❒❒ **Differentiate between dementia and delirium.**

Dementia - Irreversible impaired functioning secondary to changes/deficits in memory, spatial concepts, personality, cognition, language, motor and sensory skills, judgment, or behavior. There is no change in consciousness.

Delirium - A reversible organic mental syndrome reflecting deficits in attention, organized thinking, orientation, speech, memory, and perception. Patients are frequently confused, anxious, excited, and have hallucinations. A change in consciousness can be observed.

❒❒ **What are the major clinical findings in Alzheimer's patients?**

Memory loss, delusions, hallucinations, language impairment, loss of visual and spatial orientation, and loss of interest in life activities.

❒❒ **What is the most common cause of drug-induced hallucinations in the geriatric population?**

Propranolol.

❒❒ **What is an alternative name for an acute confusional state?**

Delirium. Diagnostic features include reduced level of consciousness, disorganized sleep-wake cycles, disturbances in attention, global cognitive impairment, and decreased or increased psychomotor activity.

❒❒ **What is the major risk of tricyclic antidepressants in the elderly?**

Orthostatic hypotension leading to falls.

❒❒ **Is violence more likely between family members or non-family members?**

Between family members. 20–50% of murders in the U.S. are committed by members of the victims' families. Spouse abuse is as high as 16% in the U.S.

❑❑ **What is the definition of domestic abuse?**

A pattern of assaultive and coercive behaviors including physical, sexual, and psychological abuse designed to gain power and control over an intimate partner.

❑❑ **Simple repetitive reactions like nail biting, thumb sucking, masturbation, or temper tantrums are manifestations of what psychological reaction in infancy?**

Adjustment reactions. These are responses to separation from the caregiver and are often associated with developmental delay.

❑❑ **What age range has the highest prevalence of drinking problems?**

18–29-year-olds have the greatest prevalence.

❑❑ **What laboratory changes are suggestive of alcoholism?**

An increase in: ALT, AST, alkaline phosphatase, amylase, bilirubin, cholesterol, GGT, LDH, MCV, PT, triglycerides, and uric acid.

A decrease in: BUN, calcium, coagulopathy, hematocrit, magnesium, phosphorus, platelet count, and protein.

❑❑ **Describe symptoms of alcohol withdrawal and their temporal relations.**

Hallucinations: Auditory, visual, and tactile; these occur 24 hours after drinking.
Autonomic hyperactivity: Tachycardia, hypertension, tremors, anxiety, and agitation; these occur 6–8 hours after drinking.
Global confusion: Occurs 1–3 days after drinking.

❑❑ **What is the most common mental illness in large cities?**

Substance abuse. Rural communities have substance abuse as well, but not in such high percentages. Incidentally opiates are predominantly a city drug while marijuana, alcohol, and amphetamines are found in both rural and urban settings.

❑❑ **A patient presents with tearing eyes, runny nose, tachycardia, hair on end, abdominal pains, nausea, vomiting, diarrhea, insomnia, pupillary dilation, and leukocytosis. What is the probable diagnosis?**

Opiate and/or opioid withdrawal. Methadone (Dolophine) are used to treat the withdrawal symptoms.

❑❑ **What is the most effective long-term treatment for alcoholism?**

Alcoholics Anonymous meetings have proven most effective in combating alcoholism permanently.

❑❑ **What is the difference between methadone and heroin?**

Methadone causes analgesia but does not cause euphoria. Habituation does occur with both drugs. The withdrawal symptoms of methadone are much less severe, but they last longer.

❑❑ **What are the 2 most common behavioral problems seen in the medical profession?**

Anxiety and depression. More cases of anxiety and depression are treated by generalists than psychiatrists.

❑❑ **Describe a patient with generalized anxiety disorder.**

Patients appear apprehensive, restless, irritable, and easily distracted. Patients may experience muscle tension and fatigue as well as various autonomic symptoms, such as palpitations, shortness of breath, chest tightness, nausea, or diffuse weakness and numbness.

❑❑ **Name a few substances that may mimic generalized anxiety when ingested.**

Nicotine, caffeine, amphetamines, cocaine, and anticholinergics. Alcohol and sedative withdrawal can also mimic this disorder.

❑❑ **What are 8 common medical causes of anxiety or anxiety attacks?**

(1) Alcohol withdrawal, (2) thyrotoxicosis, (3) caffeine, (4) stroke, (5) cardiopulmonary emergencies, (6) hypoglycemia, (7) psychosensory/psychomotor epilepsy, and (8) pheochromocytoma.

❑❑ **What is the most common cause of referral to child psychiatrists?**

Attention Deficit Hyperactivity Disorder. ADHD accounts for 30–50% of child psychiatric outpatients.

❑❑ **What are the side effects of methylphenidate (Ritalin)?**

Depression, headache, hypertension, insomnia, and abdominal pain.

❑❑ **What is the most frequent first episode of bipolar disease: mania or depression?**

Mania. Depression is rarely the first symptom. In fact, only 5–10% of patients that develop depression first go on to have manic episodes. One-third of manic patients never have a depressive episode.

❑❑ **Other than the classic mania, what can lithium be used to treat?**

Bulimia, anorexia nervosa, alcoholism in patients with mood disorders, leukocytosis in patients on antineoplastic medication, cluster headaches, and migraine headaches.

❑❑ **Should people who are physically active and taking lithium have their lithium dosage increased or decreased?**

Increased. Lithium, a salt, is excreted more than sodium during sweating.

❑❑ **T/F: A patient starting lithium will be expected to gain weight.**

True. All psychotropic medications cause weight gain, hence lithium's usefulness in treating anorexia nervosa.

❑❑ **What is the potential complication of a manic depressive who is also being treated for congestive heart failure?**

Lithium toxicity. Low salt diet and/or sodium-losing diuretics can cause lithium retention and toxicity.

❑❑ **Lithium toxicity begins at what level?**

14 mg/L. Above this level nausea, diarrhea, vomiting, rigidity, tremor, ataxia, seizures, delirium, coma, and death can all occur.

❑❑ **Why might a patient taking lithium experience polyuria?**

Long-term lithium ingestion can cause nephrogenic diabetes.

❑❑ **What is the most common clinical symptom of a patient with a borderline personality?**

Chronic boredom. Other symptoms include severe mood swings, volatile relationships, continuous and uncontrollable anger, and impulsiveness.

❑❑ **A patient presents to your office with parotid gland swelling and erosion of the enamel on her teeth. What findings might you expect to find in this patient?**

The patient described most likely has bulimia. Elevated serum amylase and hypokalemia are associated with bulimia.

❑❑ **List some common laboratory findings associated with eating disorders.**

Hyponatremia, hypokalemia, hypocalcemia, hypophosphatemia, anemia, hypoglycemia, starvation ketoacidosis, abnormal glucose tolerance, hypothyroidism due to low T3 levels, persistently elevated cortisol due to starvation, low FSH, LH and estrogens, and elevated growth hormone.

❑❑ **What are some manifestations of catatonic disorder?**

Any of the following: echolalia, echopraxia, excessive purposeless motor activity, motor immobility, extreme negativism, resistance to external instruction or movement, or peculiar involuntary movements, such as bizare posturing or grimacing.

❑❑ **Children with conduct disorder are most likely to develop what adult disorder?**

About 40% will have some pathology as adults. The most common disorder is antisocial personality disorder.

❑❑ **What is conversion disorder?**

Internal psychological conflict that manifests itself as somatic symptoms. Voluntary motor or sensory function is affected. Examples include weakness, imbalance, dysphagia, and changes in vision, hearing, or sensation. These symptoms are not feigned or intentionally produced. They are also not fully explained by medical conditions.

❑❑ **Describe dementia.**

Disturbed cognitive function resulting in impaired memory, personality, judgment, and/or language. Dementia has an insidious onset, but it may present as acute worsened mental state when the patient is facing other physical or environmental stressors.

❑❑ **Describe delirium.**

"Clouding of consciousness" resulting in disorientation, decreased alertness, and impaired cognitive function. Acute onset, visual hallucinations, and fluctuating psychomotor activity are all commonly seen. All symptoms are variable and may change over hours.

❑❑ **What are 2 major causes of dementia?**

Alzheimer's disease and multi-infarction. Demented patients may have decreased memory, cognition, language ability, judgment, and sensory and motor function. There is no change is consciousness, although personality changes do exist.

❑❑ **Name some over-the-counter and "street" drugs that may produce delirium or acute psychosis.**

Salicylates, antihistamines, anticholinergics, alcohols, phencyclidine, LSD, mescaline, cocaine, and amphetamines.

❑❑ **Name some symptoms of major depression.**

IN SAD CAGES:
- Interest
- Sleep
- Appetite
- Depressed mood
- Activity
- Guilt
- Energy
- Suicide

❑❑ **Name some vegetative symptoms.**

Loss of appetite, lack of concentration, chronic fatigue, agitation, restlessness, inability to sleep, and weight loss.

❑❑ **What is dysthymia?**

Dysthymia is a chronic disorder lasting more than 2 years. The severe symptoms of depression, such as delusions and hallucinations are absent. Patients with dysthymia have some good days, they react to their environment, and they have no vegetative signs. 10% of patients with dysthymia develop major depression.

❑❑ **Wild and abundant dreams may result from withdrawal of what drug?**

Antidepressants. Other side effects of withdrawal are anxiety, akathisia, bradykinesia, mania, and malaise.

❑❑ **What is a dystonic reaction?**

It is a very common side effect of neuroleptics seen in the ED. Muscle spasm of the tongue, face, neck, and back are seen. Severe laryngospasm and extraocular muscle spasm may occur also.

❑❑ **How do you treat a dystonic reaction?**

Diphenhydramine (Benadryl), 25–50 mg IM or IV or benztropine (Cogentin), 1–2 mg IV or PO. Remember that dystonias can recur acutely.

❏❏ What are the 5 Kubler-Ross stages?

1) Denial.
2) Anger.
3) Bargaining.
4) Depression.
5) Acceptance.

Patients may undergo all or only a few of these stages.

❏❏ A 24-year-old male presents to the ED complaining of pleuritic pain, palpitations, dyspnea, dizziness, and tingling in his arms and legs. What is the most likely cause if cardiac abnormalities are ruled out?

Hyperventilation syndrome. This is frequently associated with anxiety. The tingling is due to decreased carbonate in the blood.

❏❏ Hallucinogens affect what neurotransmitter?

Serotonin.

❏❏ What is the treatment for a "bad trip" on LSD?

Chlorpromazine can be used IM for severe or uncontrollable anxiety. Remind the patient of reality by constantly reinforcing him that his perceptions are only distortions due to the drug. This is called "talking down."

❏❏ What is the difference between malingering and a factitious disorder?

The goal of a malingerer is an external incentive such as workman's comp. The goal of a someone with factitious disorder is to enter into the sick role. Both involve voluntary faking of an illness.

❏❏ Who is at a greater risk for mood disorders: men or women?

Women by a ratio of 7:3.

❏❏ What is an extreme case of factitious disorder?

Munchausen's syndrome. These patients may actually try to cause harm to themselves (e.g., by injecting feces into their veins) and are very accepting/seeking of invasive procedures. Munchausen by proxy is another example. In this disease the patient seeks medical care for another, usually a child.

❏❏ Why is Haloperidol one of the preferred neuroleptics?

It can be used IM in emergencies, and it has few side effects. It does, however, have a high frequency of extra-pyramidal effects.

❏❏ What is the only neuroleptic that does not have tardive dyskinesia as a side effect?

Clozapine. Unfortunately, clozapine patients can develop agranulocytosis and are at a higher risk for seizures than patients on other neuroleptics. Other side effects include hypotension, anticholinergic symptoms, and over sedation.

❑❑ A non-pregnant woman taking neuroleptics complains of breast engorgement and lactation. What is the probable diagnosis?

Pseudolactation.

❑❑ What happens when one combines ETOH with a benzodiazepine?

Death due to combined respiratory depressive effects.

❑❑ Name another contraindication to benzodiazepine use.

Known hypersensitivity, acute narrow angle glaucoma, and pregnancy (especially in the first trimester).

❑❑ Why aren't mono-amine oxidase (MAO) inhibitors prescribed more frequently?

Why don't you try a tyramine-free diet sometime! Tyramine-containing substances can cause hypertensive crisis. Such foods include pickled herring, snails, chicken liver, beer, red wine, and cheese.

❑❑ Name some drugs contraindicated in a patient taking MAO inhibitors.

Toxic reactions that include excitation and hyperpyrexia can occur with meperidine (Demerol) and with dextromethorphan. The effects of indirect acting adrenergic drugs are potentiated, including ephedrine, sympathomimetic amines in cold remedies, amphetamines, cocaine, and methylphenidate (Ritalin).

❑❑ Name the 3 common MAO inhibitors (chemical and brand name).

1) Phenelzine (Nardil).
2) Isocarboxazid (Marplan).
3) Tranylcypromine (Parnate).

❑❑ What are extrapyramidal reactions?

Involuntary and spontaneous motor responses including dystonia, akathisia, and Parkinson-like syndrome.

❑❑ Obsessive compulsive disorders generally begin before what age?

25.

❑❑ What are some common obsessions?

Dirt and contamination, order and symmetry, religion and philosophy, and daily decisions. Unfortunately, compulsion does not relieve the anxiety of the obsession. Serotonin uptake inhibitors and exposure therapy have been found helpful.

❑❑ A 6-year-old boy consistently wets his pants. You tell the mother to reward dry periods with treats and praise. This will help reinforce desired behavior. What kind of conditioning is this?

Positive operant conditioning. This principle was defined by Pavlov.

❑❑ **A 20-year-old female comes to a clinic complaining of sudden episodes of palpitations, diaphoresis, lightheadedness, a fear of losing control, a sense of being choked, tremors, and paresthesias. What is the probable diagnosis?**

Panic disorder. Panic disorders need not be linked to any events. Though they are commonly associated with agoraphobia, social phobia, mitral prolapse, and late non-melancholic depression.

❑❑ **How is a patient with a PCP overdose medically treated?**

Acidify the urine with cranberry juice or NH_4Cl, give benzodiazapine, and restrain the patient.

❑❑ **Give an example for each of the following perceptual disturbances: illusion, complete auditory hallucination, functional hallucination, and extracampine hallucination.**

Illusion: A kitten is perceived as a dragon. (The patient misinterprets reality.)

Complete auditory hallucination: The patient claims to hear people talking to him when no one is around. (Clear voices are reportedly heard. They are perceived as being external to the patient.)

Functional hallucination: The patient hears voices only when cars honk their horns. (Hallucinations occur only after sensory stimulus in the same category as the hallucination.)

Extracampine hallucination: The patient can see people waving at him from the top of the Eiffel Tower—even though he is in Chicago. (Hallucinations that are external to the patients normal range of senses.)

❑❑ **Can a person get posttraumatic stress disorder (PTSD) if they did not actually witness a disturbing event?**

Yes. According to the DSM–IV, one can experience PTSD if an event, such as a violent personal assault, a serious accident, or the serious injury of a close friend or family member is learned of indirectly. PTSD can also occur after learning of a life-threatening disease in a friend or family member.

❑❑ **A 28-year-old female who was raped 6 months ago has been psychologically sound thus far. She now suddenly develops recurrent distressing flashbacks of the event, nightmares, intense fear, avoidance of all men, a diminished memory of the rape, and an exaggerated startle response. Is this woman experiencing PTSD?**

Yes. This is delayed onset PTSD. The onset of symptoms occurs at least 6 months after the provoking event.

❑❑ **What are the signs and symptoms suggestive of organic source of psychosis?**

Acute onset, disorientation, visual or tactile hallucinations, age less than 10 or older than 60, and evidence suggesting overdose or acute ingestion, such as abnormal vital signs, pupil size and reactivity (or nystagmus).

❑❑ **When are women at their greatest risk for psychiatric illness?**

The first few weeks post partum. It most often occurs in patients who are primiparous, have poor social support, or have a history of depression.

❑❑ **When does post partum psychosis begin?**

Within the first week to 10 days following childbirth. A second, smaller peak occurs 6–8 weeks post partum. This second peak correlates with the first menses post partum. Surprisingly, the risk of psychosis is lowest during pregnancy.

❑❑ **What are some characteristics of schizophrenia?**

Delusional disorder, hallucinations (usually auditory), disorganized thinking, loosening of associations, disheveled appearance, lack of insight in realizing thoughts and behavior are abnormal, onset age usually less than 40, and duration of symptoms longer than 6 months.

❑❑ **What percent of patients with schizophrenia become chronically ill?**

60–80%. Males are at a greater risk for chronic illness.

❑❑ **The onset of schizophrenia generally occurs by what age?**

80% of schizophrenics develop the disease before their early twenties. The disease is very rare after 40.

❑❑ **Separation anxiety has an average onset of what age?**

Age 9. These children fear leaving home, sleep, being alone, going to school, and losing their parents. 75% develop somatic complaints in order to avoid attending school.

❑❑ **A 30-year-old female complains of pain in her calf, headache, shooting pain when flexing her right wrist, random epigastric pain, bloating, and irregular menses, all of which cannot be explained following medical work-ups. Probable diagnosis?**

Somatization Disorder—multiple, unexplained medical symptoms involving multiple systems. In order to diagnose a patient with somatization disorder, one must have 4 or more unexplained pain symptoms. Symptoms generally begin in childhood and are full blown by the age of 30. This is more common in women than men.

❑❑ **Who is more successful at suicide: men or women?**

Women certainly try harder to kill themselves—the ratio of attempted suicides is 3:1, female: male. However, males are more successful—3:1, males:females.

❑❑ **Major depression and bipolar affective disorder account for what percentage of suicides?**

50%. Another 25% are due to substance abuse, and another 10% are attributed to schizophrenia.

❑❑ **What are predictors of a potentially violent patient?**

Male gender, history of violence, and history of substance abuse are the only reliable predictors. Cultural, educational, economic, and language barriers to effective patient/staff communication, as well as trivializing a patient or family member's concerns can increase frustrations and lower the threshold for violent episodes.

❑❑ **What mood is most frequently expressed by patients with organic brain syndrome?**

Irritability.

❑❑ **What medication can be used to relieve the extrapyramidal affects of psychotropic medications?**

Diphenhydramine, hydrochloride (Benadryl), trihexyphenidyl (Artane), and benztropine mesylate (Cogentin).

❑❑ **What are the characteristics of a labile affect?**

Rapid shifts of emotions and mood.

❑❑ **What is amnesia?**

A loss of memory from an organic or inorganic cause.

❑❑ **How do you respond to questions asked by a school-age child who is faced with a terminal illness?**

Speak to the child honestly regarding his condition and give an explanation of the diagnosis in terms he can understand. Provide reassurance that he or she will not be alone.

❑❑ **How should you respond if a terminally ill patient asks, "How much time do I have left to live?"**

Be honest and answer to the best of your knowledge. Explain that no exact time can be placed on how long a person has to live, because information is gathered from statistical information, and therefore it is only a guess.

❑❑ **What psychiatric problems are associated with violence?**

Acute schizophrenia, paranoid ideation, catatonic excitation, mania, borderline and antisocial personality disorders, delusional depression, post-traumatic stress disorder, and decompensating obsessive/compulsive disorder.

❑❑ **What are the prodromes of violent behavior?**

Anxiety, defensiveness, volatility, and physical aggression.

❑❑ **Define the following.**

Akathisia: Internal restlessness. The patient feels as if he is "jumping out of his skin." Treatment is with propranolol.

Echolali: Meaningless automatic repetition of someone else's words. This may occur immediately or even months after hearing the words.

Catalepsy: The patient maintains the same posture over a long period of time.

Waxy flexibility: The patient offers resistance to anyone trying to change his position, then gradually allows himself to be moved to a new posture, much like a clay figure.

❑❑ A patient is brought in because she believes butterflies are landing all around her. The butterflies talk to her and tell her to love everyone. She denies suicidal ideation and any desire to harm herself or others. She has no record of harming people in the past. Can this person be institutionalized against her will?

No. Unless the patient is a danger to herself or others, she cannot be confined to an institution despite questionable mental status.

❑❑ According to Holmes and Rahe, what are life's top 10 most stressful events? (Hint: taking the boards is not on the list.)

1) Death of spouse or child
2) Divorce
3) Separation
4) Institutional detention
5) Death of close family member
6) Major personal injury or illness
7) Marriage
8) Job loss
9) Marital reconciliation
10) Retirement

❑❑ What is the ratio of attempted suicides to completed suicides?

10:1.

❑❑ What is the standard of care for victims of domestic violence currently recommended by JCAHO, the AMA, and the CDC?

1) Establish a confidential system to identify DV victims.
2) Document the abuse.
3) Collect physical evidence.
4) Evaluate safety issues and potential for lethality or suicide.
5) Formulate a safety plan with the victim.
6) Advise the victim of all his/her options and resources.
7) Refer for counseling and other services, including legal assistance.
8) Coordinate with law enforcement.
9) Transport to a shelter if desired or needed.
10) Follow-up with a domestic violence advocate.

❑❑ What are some common anticholinergic medications?

Atropine, tricyclic antidepressants, antihistamines, phenothiazine and antiparkinsonian drugs.

❑❑ Describe the signs, symptoms, and ECG findings associated with lithium toxicity.

Tremor, weakness, and flattening of the T-waves, respectively.

❑❑ What is the treatment for Wernicke's encephalopathy?

Thiamine IV.

❑❑ What are the signs and symptoms of organic brain syndrome?

Onset may occur at any age. Symptoms include visual hallucinations and perceptions of the unfamiliar as familiar. Signs include mental status changes (such as disorientation, clouded sensorium, asterixis, or mild clonus) and focal neurologic signs. Vital signs are often within normal limits.

❑❑ Explain the significant features of each axis in the DSM-III official diagnostic criteria and the nomenclature for psychiatric illnesses.

Axis I: Organic brain syndromes that are caused by intoxication or a physical illness. The major psychiatric disorders include psychosis, affective disorders, and disorders of substance use.
Axis II: Personality disorders, including antisocial, schizoid, and histrionic types.
Axis III: Medical problems, such as heart disease and infections.
Axis IV: Life events that contribute to the patient's problems.
Axis V: Patient's adaptation to these problems.

❑❑ What is the most commonly abused volatile substance?

Toluene.

❑❑ A severely depressed and paranoid patient refuses to eat and a gastrostomy tube has been ordered. How would this client most likely view the tube in regards to his care?

A suspicious client may interpret a G-tube as an attack so it should be used as a last resort.

❑❑ A client taking Imipramine complains of a dry mouth and is drinking excessively. Should the nurse be concerned?

Dry mouth is a side effect of tricyclics; however, increasing the fluid intake will not relieve the symptoms and could lead to an electrolyte imbalance.

❑❑ What teaching do you need to perform in regards to the above problem?

Explain the side effects of tricyclic antidepressants. Suggest alternatives to relieve the dry mouth such as gum or ice chips.

❑❑ What is the least therapeutic affect to use around a depressed client?

Cheerfulness or gaiety. This tends to make the depressed person feel guilty and unworthy. It will not make the depressed person happier.

❑❑ What is the theory behind the interpersonal model of behavior therapy?

Behavioral changes result from stress on the individual and her/his body systems.

❑❑ What is the basic premise behind the systems model theory?

Behavior results from interaction between an individual and the environment.

❑❑ Name a possible adverse reaction to haloperidol (Haldol) involving the neurological system.

Extrapyramidal side effects.

❑❑ **A client on haloperidol (Haldol) is unable to sit still, paces around his room, and is restless. What extrapyramidal side effect is he experiencing?**

Akathisia.

❑❑ **If a paranoid client names another client on the ward as his perceived enemy, what action you take?**

Promptly report the comment to the staff and take measures to insure the safety of both clients.

❑❑ **A schizophrenic client admitted to the unit is dirty, her clothing is stained, and she has no shoes. She is confused and seems apprehensive. What should be your initial goal?**

You should always concentrate first on the patient's safety, self care needs, and health needs before any behavior goals are attempted.

❑❑ **T/F: Nonverbal communication conveys feelings more accurately than does verbal communication.**

True. It's often harder to hide true feelings nonverbally.

❑❑ **What are the major goals of a psychosocial rehabilitation program for a client with chronic mental illness?**

Teaching independent living skills, assisting with living arrangements, and setting up the patient with community resources.

❑❑ **A client has been admitted to the hospital involuntarily. What does this mean?**

The patient has been determined by a physician to be a threat to himself/herself or others.

❑❑ **A client explains that before he leaves home he checks to make sure the lights are off 52 times. What are the patient's unconscious motives for performing this activity?**

The patient is substituting emotions that are unacceptable to him with a more acceptable activity.

❑❑ **A patient refuses to have an EEG because she is concerned about electrical shock. What is your response?**

There is no risk because the EEG records the electrical activity of the brain and does not involve the use of an electrical shock.

❑❑ **Name some common clinical symptoms of a client with an organic mental disorder.**

Agnosia, sleep disturbances, decreases in both short-term and long-term memory, confusion delirium, and depression.

❑❑ **With an adolescent client, which person or authoritative group would have the most influence on her behavior?**

A group of her/his peers.

❏❏ A patient has negative feelings towards her father, but praises him constantly. What defense mechanism is at work?

Reaction formation.

❏❏ When a client attributes his own negative traits to someone else, what is this called?

Projection.

❏❏ An alcoholic client remarks he cannot remember the events of this past weekend. What is the most likely cause?

An alcoholic blackout.

❏❏ After an alcoholic has been free of alcohol, how long do tremors usually continue?

They may persist for several days or longer.

❏❏ How does disulfiram (Antabuse) help to curb the alcoholic's intake of alcohol?

It reacts with the alcohol causing a multitude of unpleasant physical symptoms proportionate to the amount of alcohol ingested.

❏❏ A patient states, "I just drink because my job is so stressful. I'm sure most people drink like me." What defense mechanism is displayed here?

Rationalization. Substituting a more acceptable reason for one's behavior.

❏❏ A client is brought to the ED after a heroin overdose. What should be your first assessment?

Assess the airway. Remember the ABC's.

❏❏ A client denies the recent use of cocaine. What physical sign could you look for to indicate inhalation of cocaine?

Red, excoriated nostrils due to local irritation, dilated pupils, nervous behavior, and increased pulse rate.

❏❏ While preparing for discharge, the chemically dependent client asks you to make arrangements for him to attend AA meetings. What is your response?

Tell the patient he needs to make his own arrangements. This encourages independence and allows the patient to take responsibility for his own recovery.

❏❏ What is the most common cause of death from a barbiturate overdose?

Respiratory failure.

❏❏ What drug is given at a non-intoxicating dose to a patient going through barbiturate withdrawal?

Pentobarbital sodium (Nembutal).

❒❒ What class of drugs is often abused for use in weight control?

Amphetamines.

❒❒ Name some of the symptoms of long-term amphetamine abuse.

Emotional lability, depression between doses, drug dependency, hallucinations, and delusions.

❒❒ A patient with anorexia nervosa is found doing sit-ups in her room. How should you handle the situation?

Interrupt the patient and direct her to another activity. Exercise is often a compulsion for the anorexic and it should not be encouraged because it could be harmful to her health.

❒❒ T/F: When a client with severe anxiety is withdrawn, you should plan activities that will increase his contact with others.

True. These clients are usually very self focused an diversion activities will help draw attention away from themselves.

❒❒ What is the ultimate nursing goal when caring for a patient with a severe anxiety disorder?

The development of adaptive coping behaviors and problem solving skills.

❒❒ A client is prescribed propanolol (Inderal) for anxiety. Should you question this order?

No. Inderal, although a common blood pressure medication, is also used to relieve the physical symptoms of anxiety.

❒❒ Why is it ineffective to make an antisocial personality feel remorseful or ashamed in order to change his behavior?

The antisocial personality is egocentric and unconcerned with his effect on others.

❒❒ A client discloses to you that he plans to kill someone when he is released. What should you do?

Tell the staff and physician immediately.

❒❒ If a patient has a obtained sense of self-awareness, attributes, defense mechanisms and behaviors, what has he gained?

Insight.

❒❒ Which developmental task follows identity and when does it usually occur?

Intimacy, which occurs in early adulthood.

❒❒ A client is admitted with depression and suicidal tendencies. What should be a priority nursing goal?

The patient will not cause harm to herself/himself.

❑❑ **Can asking a depressed client if she has suicidal thoughts or tendencies give her the idea to kill herself?**

No. Suicide is an individual decision and cannot be influenced by a nurse's questions.

❑❑ **What should you look for when assessing a client's potential for a suicide attempt?**

A sudden increase in energy level or mood. This is common prior to a suicide attempt and it symbolizes the patient having made the decision to end his life.

❑❑ **A client under the influence of cocaine is agitated, aggressive, and paranoid. What should be your first concern?**

Safety. Protect the patient from himself and others.

❑❑ **What is Tardive Dyskinesia?**

Involuntary twitching or muscle movements. Sometimes involves facial muscles with tongue-rolling movements.

❑❑ **What is dystonia?**

Uncoordinated spastic movements of the body.

❑❑ **When it is time for discharge, what should you include in your plan of care for the patient?**

Preparation for termination of the nurse-client relationship.

❑❑ **If a delusional client refuses to attend activities and spends all his time alone, should you ignore this behavior and give him time to make contact with others at his own pace?**

No. Leaving a client alone, especially one who is delusional, will allow him to further isolate and withdraw into himself. Encourage him to participate with others to reinforce reality.

❑❑ **What would be your first course of action for the above client?**

Initiate brief one-on-one contacts with the patient in his own room.

❑❑ **T/F: To encourage a patient who refuses to speak to begin talking, you should use hand signals.**

False. This is often ineffective and may encourage the patient to continue his behavior. Using non-demanding open-ended questions will give the patient the opportunity to speak when he is ready.

❑❑ **What property of fluphenazine decanoate (Prolixin) makes it the drug of choice for many schizophrenics?**

It only needs to be given once every 2-4 weeks.

❑❑ **While a client is on fluphenazine (Prolixin), why should you monitor the patient's weight, WBC count, and blood pressure?**

Edema, blood dyscrasias, and blood pressure fluctuations are all possible side effects of this drug.

❑❑ **When a client with a chronic schizophrenia, living independently, reports he is beginning to hear voices, what should you check in regards to the patient's medication?**

Check on the patient's past record of medication administration to spot any non-compliance or missed doses.

❑❑ **What determines a client's discharge from an involuntary admission?**

Medical or legal approval.

❑❑ **What would be the best course of action to take when you observe a patient performing obsessive-compulsive behaviors?**

Allow the patient to perform the behavior if it is not harmful to the patient. Denying the patient behavior before he is ready to stop could lead to an increase in both anxiety and agitation.

❑❑ **A patient asks you to help prepare his will. What would be your best response?**

A nurse is not qualified to perform this legal task. Tell the patient to seek legal advice.

❑❑ **For a confused client, what type of interventions take priority?**

Those that promote safety, prevent injury, and maintain the patient's quality of life.

❑❑ **An intoxicated client is admitted. What is the best method to promote alcohol metabolism in the body?**

Allow the patient to sleep it off. EtOH is metabolized at a slow and steady rate.

❑❑ **The physician orders lorazepam (Ativan) and chlordiazepoxide (Librium) for a patient experiencing EtOH withdrawal. Why?**

These medications ease withdrawal symptoms by providing sedation and relieving anxiety.

❑❑ **What is a dry drunk?**

A client who has stopped alcohol consumption, but continues to use many of the defense mechanisms associated with alcoholism.

❑❑ **Describe some milder symptoms of an alcohol-disulfuram reaction.**

Flushing, throbbing in the head and neck due to vasodilatation, nausea, diaphoresis, palpitations, hyperventilation, and headache.

❑❑ **What factors usually differentiate an alcoholic from a social drinker?**

The alcoholic has an inability to get along in his relationships at work and at home due to his alcohol consumption.

❑❑ When a client is in denial, should you force the patient to face the facts as a way of initiating the therapy process?

No. Breaking a client's defenses before he is ready could lead to mental disorganization and depression.

❑❑ The doctor orders chlorpromazine (Thorazine) 100 mg every 4 hours PRN for agitation in a client experiencing delirium tremens from EtOH withdrawal. Why should this be questioned?

Chlorpromazine reduces the seizure threshold in a client who is already at a high risk for seizures due to CNS irritability.

❑❑ A client admitted to the ED with symptoms of increased heart rate, dilated pupils, increased blood pressure, and increased temperature, suggests what type of substance abuse?

Stimulant abuse.

❑❑ A heroin addict experiencing withdrawal symptoms has nausea, vomiting, and diarrhea. Are these early or late signs of withdrawal?

Late.

❑❑ A patient begins methadone therapy and you note shallow respirations at the rate of 8. What could this indicate?

Methadone toxicity.

❑❑ A patient recovering from chemical dependency remarks he feels overwhelmed with the thought of being sober the rest of his life. What common recovery principle could you use to ease the patient's anxiety?

"One day at a time." Looking at recovery more than one day at a time can be overwhelming. Referring the patient to AA will help get the patient support from other addicts and help him learn the principles of recovery.

❑❑ A client is brought to the ED after consuming barbiturates and alcohol. Why would you be concerned with this chemical combination?

Taking alcohol and barbiturates together have an additive effect, thus increasing the depressant effect.

❑❑ Approximately 2-3 days into the withdrawal from barbiturates, you should be prepared for what potentially fatal occuence?

Generalized convulsions.

❑❑ What purpose does pentobarbital (Nembutal) serve when given to the addict going through barbiturate withdrawal?

It can help prevent the possibility of fatal seizures.

❑❑ Name some of the physical manifestations of anorexia nervosa.

Rapid weight loss, bradycardia, hypotension, and cold sensitivity.

❒❒ **What is the goal of hospitalization for anorexia nervosa?**

Stabilize the patient's weight and facilitate entry into outpatient care.

❒❒ **What is the difference between neurotic and normal anxiety?**

Neurotic anxiety is out of proportion to the cause whereas normal anxiety has an easily traceable stimuli and decreases over time.

❒❒ **Why is alprazolam (Xanax) used on a short-term basis as a treatment for anxiety?**

Physical and psychological dependence as well as tolerance can occur.

❒❒ **A new client is admitted to the psych unit with a diagnosis of non-specific personality disorder. What is the best method to assess baseline behaviors of this client: in isolation or on the unit?**

Observation on the unit will yield the best information because you can assess the patient's reactions to others and his environment in an objective manner.

❒❒ **When a client tries to evoke feelings of anger or a negative response from you, what is your best action?**

Do not respond to the patient. Any response by you may reinforce the negative behavior.

❒❒ **It has been found that a client's antisocial behavior stems from his resentment towards his sister. Should this be directly pointed out to the patient?**

The therapy will be more effective if the patient is assisted in discovering this for himself.

❒❒ **What is endogenous depression?**

Depression that is biochemical in nature and not related to an outside stressor.

❒❒ **What is a possible urinary system complication resulting from the use of amitriptyline hydrochloride?**

Urinary retention.

❒❒ **A client has a mental illness and is brought to the ED by her family, who wish the patient to be admitted. The patient refuses admission and wants to go home. What will determine the patient's need for admission?**

The patient must be a threat to herself or others or be unable to take care of herself in order to be admitted involuntarily, even if the family desires admission.

❒❒ **An elderly client is brought to the hospital with dementia due to a cerebral abscess. How is this dementia classified?**

As an organic mental disorder.

❑❑ **Is it wise to allow the elderly client with an organic mental disorder to reminisce about her past over and over?**

Yes. Reminiscing can help reduce depression and lessen the patient's feelings of isolation and loneliness.

❑❑ **When admitting a patient for alcohol detoxification, why should you inquire about the amount of alcohol consumed over the last 24-48 hours?**

To help determine the severity of the withdrawal.

❑❑ **When do alcoholic hallucinations usually occur?**

After ending or reducing heavy drinking. The hallucinations are usually auditory.

❑❑ **What medication is given to alcoholics to curb impulsive drinking?**

Disulfiram (Antabuse).

❑❑ **An alcoholic client is experiencing delirium tremens. To prevent potential injury to himself, he is retrained and left with an attendant in a quiet room. Is this appropriate?**

Unless the patient is extremely violent, it would be best not to restrain him. This could increase his anxiety. Having someone in the room is best for the patient's safety, especially when he is experiencing hallucinations.

❑❑ **A drug abuser with a history of heroin injection should be encouraged to be tested for what diseases?**

HIV and Hepatitis.

❑❑ **What is a drawback to outpatient methadone therapy?**

It is effective at low doses, so the patient may use what he/she needs and sell the rest.

❑❑ **How can methadone be administered to an outpatient to ensure compliance and prevent selling on the streets?**

Administer in liquid form under direct supervision.

❑❑ **What factor best measures the patient's success in recovery?**

The number of chemically free days. The longer the patient is sober, the greater chance she/he has of remaining sober.

❑❑ **What is the definition of drug tolerance?**

It requires increasingly larger doses to achieve the same desired effect.

❑❑ **Name some of the severe symptoms of barbiturate withdrawal.**

Postural hypotension, psychosis, hyperthermia, and seizures.

❑❑ **For a client admitted with anorexia nervosa, you should initially focus on what aspect of patient care?**

Nutritional status. Self-starvation can be life-threatening, so weight gain should be the first priority rather than concentrating on therapy to change the patient's behavior.

❑❑ **Upon admission, a patient is perspiring, tachypneic, complaining of vertigo, and has heart palpitations. If cardiac dysfunction is ruled out, what is the most likely psychological cause?**

Acute anxiety attack.

❑❑ **The patient on chlordiazepoxide (Librium) should avoid what foods?**

Alcoholic beverages due to additive effects.

❑❑ **What is the most important message to convey to a client when disciplining unacceptable behavior?**

Although the patient's behavior is not acceptable, the patient as a person is accepted.

❑❑ **The alcoholic who craves a drink is best helped by what type of intervention?**

Group support from other alcoholics is even more effective than one-on-one staff support.

❑❑ **Describe the moderate-to-severe symptoms of an alcohol-disulfiram reaction.**

Vomiting, dyspnea, hypotension, vertigo, syncope, confusion, respiratory depression, convulsions, coma, and death.

❑❑ **The family of an alcoholic doesn't believe their son drinks too much or that his loss of 4 jobs in 4 months is a result of alcohol abuse. What defense mechanism is at work here?**

Denial.

❑❑ **The physician orders naloxone (Narcan) for a client who has overdosed on heroin. What effect will this have?**

Reversal of the heroin effects: increased heart rate, increased blood pressure, and increased level of consciousness.

❑❑ **After administering Narcan, a patient becomes more alert and vital signs have stabilized. Should you be at ease now that the narcotic effects have been reversed?**

No. A reversal of the Narcan effect and a return of the symptoms related to narcotic use may still occur. Narcan is very short-acting.

❑❑ **Should an HIV-positive patient be placed in a private room?**

Only if the presence of another infection warrants it, or if the immunocompromised status of the patient deems it necessary to prevent the exposure of an infectious agent from another patient.

❑❑ **Why is a heroin addict prone to diseases such as Hepatitis, pneumonia and TB?**

Poor sanitation, malnutrition, needle sharing, and an unhealthful lifestyle.

❑❑ **What is drug habituation?**

Mild dependence on a drug without addiction.

❑❑ **A client is sluggish, irritable, has difficulty walking, slurred speech, and impaired judgment. If no alcohol is present on his breath, what substance could the patient be abusing?**

A barbiturate, opiate, or benzodiazepine.

❑❑ **Name a simple way to decrease the respiratory rate in a client that is hyperventilating.**

Have the patient breathe into a paper bag.

❑❑ **A patient is prescribed buspirone (Buspar) 10 mg at HS PRN. Why should this order be questioned?**

Buspar is not effective when given PRN. Therapeutic effects take 7-10 days, and full effects are not seen for 3-4 weeks.

❑❑ **What are the personality characteristics of a patient with an antisocial personality disorder?**

Lack of guilt, sorrow, or remorse for her/his actions.

❑❑ **Does peristalsis increase or decrease when epinephrine is released by the body?**

Decreases.

❑❑ **What are some of the common characteristics of an abusive family?**

An unbalanced power ratio, stereotypical role-playing, dysfunctional expression of feelings, strict boundaries, lack of empathy, substance abuse, and a history of family violence.

❑❑ **T/F: Low self esteem is a common trait among abuse victims.**

True.

❑❑ **A client with AIDS lies in bed all day, refuses to eat, and will not communicate with the staff. What stage of grief is he in?**

Depression.

❑❑ **When should restraints be discontinued on a client?**

When subjective and objective assessments indicate an absence of aggression.

❑❑ **When can medication be forced upon a client?**

Only if the patient poses a threat to the self or others without it.

❑❑ T/F: A patient suffering from a phobia should be forced to confront his anxiety.

False. This could cause extreme panic. Gradual exposure to the phobia is preferred.

❑❑ What is the best approach to use when dealing with an antisocial personality?

Limit-setting on behaviors.

❑❑ A client is admitted who has trouble expressing his anger. Before the patient's first outburst occurs, what should you discuss with the patient?

Appropriate actions for the patient when he begins to feel angry.

❑❑ Name some of the symptoms of the autonomic nervous system's response to epinephrine.

Increased blood pressure, increased respiratory rate, muscle tension, dilated pupils, increased heart rate, decreased peristalsis.

❑❑ A battered wife is advised by a nurse to leave her husband. Why is this not appropriate?

The patient should not be told to leave her spouse or given any unsolicited advice. Coercing the patient takes away responsibility for her own actions and could lead to resentment towards the nurse.

❑❑ When a client is admitted with a psycho-physiological disorder related to anxiety, what type of activities should you promote for the patient?

Those that will promote rest, are of low anxiety, and involve relaxation techniques.

❑❑ Before caring for terminally ill clients, you must examine what aspect of yourself in order to be the most effective?

Your views and feelings towards mortality.

❑❑ A client with a history of aggressive behavior is displaying signs of agitation. How should you handle the situation?

Encourage the patient to discuss his feelings while pointing out his behavior and trying to avert an aggressive outburst. Don't assume the patient is agitated and take defensive action unless it is warranted.

❑❑ Amitriptyline 75 mg q HS and phenelzine (Nardil) 15 mg t.i.d. are ordered. What would be a nursing priority before administering these medications?

Call the physician to clarify the order. These medications are usually not ordered together.

❑❑ For a patient with an organic mental disorder, you should create what type of environment?

A safe, simple environment to help with his/her orientation.

❑❑ A patient who is a perfectionist, exercises constantly, and shows self-destructive tendencies such

as self-starvation most likely has what disorder?

Anorexia nervosa.

❑❑ **Why are isolation, medications, or warning others not the best long-term treatment plan for a patient who has angry outbursts?**

While these interventions may help for the short term, they do not place any responsibility on the patient for her/his own behavior and thus will be ineffective in modifying the patient's behavior for the long term.

❑❑ **For an aggressive client, what purpose does anger usually serve?**

It is a defense mechanism or a way of dealing with a situation. It can protect the patient, make him/her feel more powerful or energized, but this does not last and angry outbursts may occur with increasing frequency over time.

❑❑ **What information should you give a battered client who refuses to press charges before she leaves?**

A list of resources and phone numbers for battered women. Just because the patient refused treatment does not mean you should not give the patient needed resources.

❑❑ **Haloperidol (Haldol) 100 mg PO or IM every 4 hours is ordered for a client. What would be the nursing action if the patient is agitated?**

Call first to confirm the dose. Normal dosing is 5-100 mg daily.

❑❑ **Administration of an MAO inhibitor too soon after stopping tricyclic therapy can cause what side effects?**

Hypertension and hyperpyrexia.

❑❑ **What is the best snack for a patent with anorexia nervosa?**

One that is high in both calories and proteins.

❑❑ **For the manipulative client, what type of nursing goals will produce acceptable behaviors?**

Those that involve limit-setting and positive reinforcement for the correct behavior.

❑❑ **When a client has an angry outburst and handles it appropriately, how should you respond?**

Positively reinforce the patient's behavior.

❑❑ **What is the best indicator of a client's potential for violence?**

Past history.

❑❑ **What are some of the possible characteristics of the abuser in an abusive relationship?**

Alcoholic, low self esteem, need for control and power, a history of family abuse, and a lack of empathy.

❑❑ **Name personality traits associated with ulcerative colitis.**

Obsessive-compulsive, perfectionist, inflexible, difficulty in showing emotions, and obstinate.

❑❑ **A client is in 4-point restraints. What are some nursing goals for this client?**

The patient must be monitored at all times in order to provide a safe environment and prevent injury to the patient. Allowing the patient to change position, providing a means of elimination and nutrition, providing sensory stimulation, monitoring circulation to the restrained extremities, and preserving skin integrity under the restraints are all nursing goals. Of course, working towards getting the patient out of restraints is also a goal.

❑❑ **You observe a patient responding to a visual hallucination and the patient asks you if you see it too. How should you react?**

Tell the patient that you believe that he does see something, but that you do not. Do not "play along" with the patient's hallucination.

❑❑ **How long does it take for the therapeutic effects of MAO inhibitors to be seen after the first dose?**

4 weeks.

❑❑ **What is a conversion reaction?**

The transfer of unacceptable feelings into a physical symptom that has no identifiable cause.

❑❑ **What hormone is released in the body when one becomes angry.**

Epinephrine.

❑❑ **A patient responds sarcastically when asked to perform a unit activity. Of what emotion is sarcasm an expression?**

Anger.

❑❑ **Abused women often feel alone and ashamed. What resource could you suggest for this patient?**

A support group for battered women.

❑❑ **When assessing a client who was admitted after having suffered physical abuse from her husband, with what should the nurse first be concerned?**

The safety of the patient in regards to any immediate danger and treating the patient for any physical injuries. Dealing with psychological issues comes after safety and physical well-being.

❑❑ **What is confabulation?**

An unconscious behavior used to hide memory loss by replacing it with a fabrication.

❑❑ **What foods should be avoided while on MAO inhibitors?**

Foods that contain tyramine.

❑❑ **A client does not remember witnessing her father's murder. What is this defense mechanism called?**

Repression.

❑❑ **When dealing with a client who has a terminal illness, how should you respond when the patient expresses hopelessness in regards to her future?**

Always allow the patient to express her feelings so she can deal with them effectively. Do not offer pat answesr or give false hope.

❑❑ **A psychiatric client voluntarily admitted wishes to be discharged, but her physician denies this request. What would be the physician's reasoning?**

The patient has been found to be a danger to herself and/or others and the physician may legally hold the patient for 72 hours.

❑❑ **What side effect could occur when the patient on MAO inhibitors drinks red wine?**

Hypertensive or hyperpyretic crisis.

❑❑ **What is the term for the projection of thoughts or feelings onto someone else?**

Transference.

❑❑ **A patient on an MAO inhibitor complains of headache and neck stiffness. Should you be concerned?**

These symptoms could indicate the beginnings of a hypertensive crisis. Withhold the next dose of medication until the physician is notified and monitor the patient's vital signs.

❑❑ **A new client is admitted to the unit and she refuses to speak to anyone. How should the nurse approach the patient?**

Use open-ended questions that focus on the expression of one's feelings, but do not push the patient to respond. Do not let the patient isolate herself since this could cause further regression.

❑❑ **For an anorexic client, what is the subconscious reason for denying her body food?**

It is usually a means of controlling anxiety stemming from a variety of factors. These can include autonomy, identity, and parental conflicts.

❑❑ **Why is a patient instructed not to abruptly stop taking anti-psychotic medication?**

Nausea or seizures can result from the abrupt withdrawal of these medications.

❑❑ **Manipulative behavior is usually the result of a lack of what?**

Trust. A manipulative client cannot trust her/his own feelings and therefore cannot trust others.

❑❑ A client is admitted in the manic phase of his bipolar disorder and is busily attending to several activities. Why should you be cautious when trying to redirect the patient's activities to the unit's routine?

Bipolar clients are prone to erratic and unpredictable behavior especially when challenged.

❑❑ A client admitted to the psychiatric unit has been overeating and has been found vomiting soon after she eats. What is most likely her diagnosis?

Bulimia.

❑❑ When admitting a client with an eating disorder, what is your first priority?

Physical and nutritional status.

❑❑ A client states he would be better off dead. How should you respond?

You should ask questions to determine the seriousness of the patient's threat, and encourage the patient to further express his emotions.

❑❑ A client with anorexia states she hates being in the hospital and wants to go home. You try to comfort her by saying, "Don't worry, you will feel better tomorrow." Is this appropriate?

No, because it gives false reassurances to the patient and does not address her real feelings of wanting to go home.

❑❑ When a client is becoming verbally and physically abusive, what should you do before using physical restraints or chemical interventions?

Try setting limits verbally.

❑❑ When assessing an abused child, what would you expect his emotional level to be?

Very passive with little showing of emotion and little response to pain.

❑❑ What should you look for when assessing a depressed client's readiness to return home?

Signs that the patient is ready to take responsibility for his own well being, such as continuing his treatment on an outpatient basis.

❑❑ An abused child is assigned the same primary nurse every day. How will this benefit the patient?

It will promote trust and provide continuity of care.

❑❑ A patient with anorexia nervosa should always be monitored for what behavior?

Self-destructive behaviors such as not eating or over-exercising.

❏❏ When a patient with an antisocial personality disorder refuses to perform a set task, how should you respond?

Continue to enforce the rules and set limits on behavior.

❏❏ A client with an obsessive-compulsive disorder brushes her hair at least 100 times a day. Should you allow the patient to engage in this behavior?

Yes, but monitor her hair brushing and set limits on the behavior. Prohibiting the behavior entirely could cause too much anxiety.

❏❏ A client with an antisocial personality disorder wants to skip group because he is busy watching TV. How should you handle this?

Explain to the patient why he will not be able to continue watching TV and send him to the group. Always set limits and give an appropriate explanation.

❏❏ A patient with an organic mental disorder is often unable to perform basic self-care tasks. What should you include in her care plan regarding this client?

Assist the patient in performing self-care tasks and encourage the patient to perform as much self-care as possible.

❏❏ A patient with a bipolar disorder in the manic phase is most likely to have what type of eating habits?

Decreased appetite. The manic client usually doesn't slow down long enough to eat and intake should be monitored closely.

❏❏ When a client comes to you upset or in distress about an event, what should you do?

Give support and be empathetic. This will validate the patient's feelings and allow an opportunity to continue talking about the patient's situation.

❏❏ Since losing her job, a 30-year-old female has been unable to leave the house because of palpitations, sweating, shortness of breath, and a feeling of impending doom. What is she most likely suffering from?

Panic attacks.

❏❏ When a client comes in to the ED suffering from a panic attack, you state, "You are experiencing panic attacks. If you relax and stop drinking coffee, they will decrease over time." Is this response appropriate?

No. Telling the patient she is having a panic attack might help her gain insight into her problem, but if she is not ready to hear that her problem is psychological rather than physical, this could be offensive.

❏❏ What is an important nursing component of any nursing care plan?

Diagnosis, goals, interventions, and evaluation

❑❑ After the recent loss of her husband, a patient states, "Why couldn't those doctors save his life, they must be incompetent!" What stage of grief is the patient experiencing?

Anger.

❑❑ Can meperidine (Demerol) be given to a patient on MAO inhibitors?

No, it can cause death.

❑❑ A patient with Alzheimer's having difficulty with memory and emotions is said to be in what stage of the disease?

Stage 1.

❑❑ What are some of the characteristics of Stage 3 Alzheimer's?

Memory loss, confusion, wandering, inability to understand or express the spoken word, echolalia, and an inability to maintain physiological functions.

❑❑ For a patient taking Lithium, what food should be monitored closely in order to avoid toxicity?

Sodium.

❑❑ What types of foods are considered high in tyramine?

Those that have been smoked, aged, pickled, or fermented.

❑❑ Would you expect a patient in Stage 1 Alzheimer's to have total memory loss?

No. Recent memory loss is more common.

❑❑ You ask a client to explain the phrase "A rolling stone gathers no moss." What are you assessing?

Abstract thinking.

❑❑ You ask a patient why he thinks he has been admitted to the hospital. What does this assessment indicate?

Insight.

❑❑ What would be a good indicator that a client has moved through the grieving process?

A willingness to return to social activities and make plans for the future.

❑❑ If a patient is actively hallucinating, what information should you gather?

If the hallucination is telling the patient to harm anyone, be it the patient, himself, or others.

❑❑ A client misses her Lithium dose. Should she double the next dose?

No. This could put the patient at risk for toxicity. Have her continue taking the doses as scheduled.

❑❑ **T/F: Delirium often has a physiological rather than a psychological basis.**

True. Factors such a hypoxia or medications can cause delirium.

❑❑ **A paranoid schizophrenic believes you are the receiver for radio waves that invade his brain. How should you respond?**

Re-direct the patient to an activity in reality. Avoid reinforcing the patient's delusions by concentrating on them.

❑❑ **The wife of a deceased client wants to see her husband's body before the funeral home comes. Why is it important for you to honor this request?**

It allows the individual to start the grieving process.

❑❑ **For a patient with dementia who has a history of wandering, what should you include in the plan of care?**

Providing a safe environment for the patient by providing constant supervision.

❑❑ **Why are restrains not used as often for elderly clients with dementia?**

The use of restraints can actually increase the incidence of injury such as vasoconstriction, nerve damage, and abrasions. They can also cause more confusion, frustration, and decrease the will to live.

❑❑ **The family of a 60-year-old widow is concerned because their mother is taking the death of her husband so well after he died of a long bout with terminal cancer. How should you respond?**

Explain that the long illness could have allowed the wife to become prepared for her husband's death and she may have experienced some anticipatory grieving already. Don't assume that the widow is in denial of her husband's death without further evidence.

❑❑ **How long does it take lithium carbonate to reach it's therapeutic level?**

2 weeks.

❑❑ **A client exhibiting manic behavior is placed on lithium carbonate and chlorpromazine (Thorazine). What is the function of chlorpromazine in this case?**

Most likely to control the manic behavior until the lithium carbonate reaches its therapeutic level.

❑❑ **A schizophrenic states she is from a distant planet and the FBI is out to capture and study her. You ask, "Really, what planet are you from?" What is wrong with this response?**

It reinforces the patient's delusion and does nothing to help the patient in giving it up.

❑❑ **A client with dementia is admitted to a nursing home. What should be a priority for the nursing care plan?**

To provide a safe environment for the patient.

❑❑ **A confused client is brought to the ED after wandering outside, without proper attire in a wind chill of 10 degrees below zero. What should be your initial nursing actions?**

Assess and attend to the patient's medical needs.

❑❑ **A client expresses sadness over the death of her friend. You state, "I can see how upsetting this is for you." Why is this a good response?**

It validates and supports the patient's feelings.

❑❑ **According to Maslow's hierarchy of needs, which needs have the highest priority?**

Physiologic needs (air, water, food, shelter, sex, activity, and comfort).

❑❑ **What is a fugue state?**

It is a dissociative state in which a person leaves familiar surroundings, assumes a new identity and develops amnesia about the previous identity.

❑❑ **What term is used for an alcoholic who achieves sobriety?**

Recovering alcoholic (because there is no cure for alcoholism at present).

❑❑ **What is the most common symptom of Alzheimer's disease?**

Memory loss.

❑❑ **To what does "flight of ideas" refer?**

An alteration in thought processes characterized by skipping from one topic to another unrelated topic.

❑❑ **What is la belle indifference?**

The lack of concern for a profound disability such as blindness or paralysis that may occur in a patient with a conversion disorder.

❑❑ **What is the highest treatment priority in a patient with anorexia nervosa?**

Correction of nutritional and electrolyte imbalance.

❑❑ **What are early signs and symptoms of alcohol withdrawal?**

Anxiety, anorexia, tremors, and insomnia (they may begin up to 8 hours after the last alcohol intake).

❑❑ **What is echolalia?**

Parrot-like repetition of another person's words or phrases. It commonly occurs in schizophrenia.

❑❑ **In a psychiatric setting, what is the purpose of seclusion?**

It promotes therapeutic limit setting, reduces overwhelming environmental stimulation, protects the patient from self-injury or injury to others, and prevents damage to hospital property.

❑❑ **When is seclusion used?**

It is used for patients who do not respond to less restricted interventions and it helps control external behavior until the patient can assume self-control.

❑❑ **What is a compulsion?**

An irresistible urge to perform an irrational act, such as walking in a clockwise circle before leaving a room.

❑❑ **What are the compocnets of self-esteem needs?**

Feelings of self-worth, self-respect, independence, self-reliance, and dignity.

❑❑ **What are the components of love and belonging needs?**

Affiliation, affection, and intimacy.

❑❑ **What is sublimation?**

The channeling of unacceptable impulses into socially acceptable behavior.

❑❑ **What is displacement?**

The transfer of unacceptable feelings to a more acceptable object.

❑❑ **What is regression?**

A retreat to an earlier developmental stage.

❑❑ **Describe a histrionic personality disorder.**

An excessive attention seeking and emotional behavior by people who are seeking praise and approval from others.

❑❑ **For ECT to be effective, how many treatments should a patient receive?**

6-12 treatments at a rate of 2-3 per week.

❑❑ **What is circumstantiality?**

A disturbance in associate thought and speech patterns in which a person gives unnecessary minute details and digresses into inappropriate thoughts which delay communication of central ideas or goal achievement.

❑❑ **What are the characteristics of a labile effect?**

Rapid shifts of emotions and mood.

❑❑ **What is amnesia?**

Loss of memory from an organic or inorganic cause.

❑❑ **T/F: A patient who is admitted involuntarily to a psychiatric hospital may sign out against medical advice.**

False.

❑❑ **What is the order of Maslow's hierarchy of needs?**

Physiologic, safety and security, love and belonging, self-esteem and recognition, and self-actualization.

❑❑ **What does somnambulism mean?**

Sleep walking.

❑❑ **What mood is most frequently experienced by a patient with organic brain syndrome?**

Irritability.

❑❑ **What medication can be used to relieve the extrapyramidal adverse affect of psychotropic medications?**

Diphenhydramine hydrochloride, trihexyphenidyl (Artane), and benztropine mesylate (Cogentin).

❑❑ **How often should lithium levels be checked?**

Every 6-8 weeks.

❑❑ **What is the drug of choice for treating attention deficit disorder in hyperactive children?**

Methylphenidate hydrochloride (Ritalin).

❑❑ **What is the most effective way to control manipulative behavior?**

Set limits.

❑❑ **What is the primary purpose of psychotropic medications?**

To decrease the patient's symptoms sufficiently to allow participation in therapy.

❑❑ **What is the first step in managing a drug overdose or drug toxicity?**

Establish and maintain an airway.

❑❑ **A patient presents with hallucinations, confabulation, amnesia and disturbances of orientation. What disorder does he have?**

Korsakoff's syndrome.

❒❒ **What is the most common psychiatric disorder?**

Depression.

❒❒ **A patient presents with hypervigilance, hostility and suspicion towards others. What personality disorder is he exhibiting?**

Paranoid personality disorder.

❒❒ **What are the adverse reactions to tricyclic antidepressants?**

Anxiety, hypomania, orthostatic hypotension, tremors, seizures, weight gain, and tachycardia. In overdose TCA's can cause hypertension, shock, malignant cardiac arrythmias, seizures and death.

BIBLIOGRAPHY

BOOKS/ARTICLES:

Bakerman, S. ABCs of Interpretive Laboratory Data (2nd Ed.). Greenville: Interpretive Laboratory Data, Inc., 1984.

Berkow, R. The Merck Manual (15th Ed.). Rahway: Merck Sharp & Dohme Research Laboratories, 1987.

Bork, K. Diagnosis and Treatment of Common Skin Diseases. Philadelphia: W.B. Saunders Company, 1988.

Dambro, M.R. Griffith's 5 Minute Clinical Consult. Williams and Wilkins, 1996.

Frye, C. Frye's 2000 Nursing Bullets (3rd Ed.). Springhouse, Pennsylvania. Springhouse Corporation, 1994.

Harrison, T.R. Principles of Internal Medicine (11th Ed.). New York: McGraw-Hill Book Company, 1987.

Harwood-Nuss, A. The Clinical Practice of Emergency Medicine (2nd Ed.). Philadelphia: J.B. Lippincott Company, 1996.

Hoppenfeld, S. Physical Examination of the Spine and Extremities. Norwalk: Appleton-Century-Crofts, 1976.

Nettina, S.M. The Lippincott Manual of Nursing Practice (6th Ed.). Philadelphia: J.B. Lippincott Company, 1996.

Perkins, E.S. An Atlas of Diseases of the Eye (3rd Ed.). London: Churchill Livingstone, 1986.

Phipps, W.J., Cassmeyer, V.L., Sands, J.K. Medical Surgical Nursing: Concepts and Clinical Practice (5th Ed.). St. Louis: Mosby Year Book, 1995.

Physicians' Desk Reference (50th Ed.). Oradell: Medical Economics Company Inc., 1996.

Pillitteri, A. Maternal and Child Health Nursing: Care of the Childbearing and Childrearing Family (2nd Ed.). Philadelphi J.B. Lippincott Company, 1995.

Plantz, SH. Emergency Medicine PreTest, Self-Assessment and Review, McGraw- Hill, 1990.

Plantz, S.H., Adler, J.N., Emergency Medicine Pearls of Wisdom. (4th Ed.). Boston Medical Publishing, 1997.

Rosen, P. Emergency Medicine Concepts and Clinical Practice (3rd Ed.). St. Louis: Mosby Year Book, 1992.

Rowe, R.C. The Harriet Lane Handbook (11th Ed.). Chicago: Year Book Medical Publishers, Inc., 1987.
Shives, L.R. Basic Concepts of Psychiatric-Mental Health Nursing (4th Ed.). Philadelphia: J.B. Lippincott

Company, 1997.

Stedman, T.L. Illustrated Stedman's Medical Dictionary (24th Ed.). Baltimore: Williams & Wilkins, 1982.

Stewart, C.E. Environmental Emergencies. Baltimore: Williams and Wilkins, 1990.

Textbook of Pediatric Advanced Life Support. Dallas: American Heart Association, 1988.

Tintinalli, J.E. Emergency Medicine A Comprehensive Study Guide (4th Ed.). New York: McGraw-Hill, Inc., 1996.

Whaley, L.F., Wong, D.L. Whaley & Wong's Essentials of Pediatric Nursing (5th Ed.). St. Louis: Mosby Year Book, 1997.